Dear Uncle Dick,
I hope you enjoy this book. It's not your typical reading but I know you have an interest in oriental medicine. Who knows where it will lead you.
Love,
Don

The Natural Healer's Acupressure Handbook, Volume I: Basic G-Jo

Other books you will find useful and enjoy by this author, published by Falkynor Books:

The Natural Healer's Acupressure Handbook, Volume II:
  Advanced G-Jo
First Aid Using Simple Remedies
How to Heal Yourself Using Foot Acupressure
  (Foot Reflexology)
How to Heal Yourself Using Hand Acupressure
  (Hand Reflexology)
The G-Jo Institute Manual of Medicinal Herbs
The G-Jo Institute Manual of Vitamins & Minerals
A Way of Eating for Pleasure and Health
The Tao of Health: The Way of Total Well-Being

Available titles in this author's **ACUGENICS** series:

The G-Jo Institute Permanent Weight Loss Program
The G-Jo Institute Stop Smoking Soon Program
The G-Jo Institute Arthritis Self-Health Program
The G-Jo Institute Sexual Pleasure Enhancement Program
The G-Jo Institute Meditative Relaxation Program

Recorded programs by this author:

ACUGENICS : Beat Stress in Five Minutes or Less!
  (Available on 33 L.P. or cassette tape)
Basic G-Jo Home Workshop (on cassette tape)

CONTACT:

The G-Jo Institute
Post Office Box 8060,
Hollywood, Florida 33084

(Retail and direct mail
  customers — send SASE
  for free literature and
  current catalog)

Falkynor Books
Post Office Box 290057,
Davie, Florida 33329

(Bookstores and jobbers)

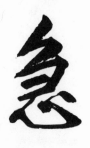

The Natural Healer's Acupressure Handbook, Volume I: Basic G-Jo

by Michael Blate

foreword by Barry Sultanoff, M.D.

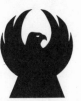

THE SPECIAL G-JO INSTITUTE EDITION
FALKYNOR BOOKS
Fort Lauderdale, Florida

to my family—Martin, Sylvia, Laurie and Keith—
for their unending patience;
and to Sri Sathya Sai Baba,
the diamond of the universe . . .

Copyright©1976, 1977, 1983 by Michael Blate
All rights reserved, including the right to reproduce this book or
portions thereof in any form.
First edition published in 1976 under the title *The G-Jo Handbook*.
Next edition published in 1977 under the title *The Natural Healer's
Acupressure Handbook*.

Cover design by MangoMedia! (Davie, Florida)

Library of Congress Cataloging in Publication Data

Blate, Michael, 1938-
    The natural healer's acupressure handbook, volume I: basic G-Jo.
    Bibliography: p.195
    1. Shiatsu. 2. Medicine, Chinese. I. Title.
RM723.S5B57   615'.822   76-45282
The G-Jo Institute special enlarged edition
Falkynor Books
ISBN Casebound edition: 0-916878-28-7
Expanded edition (supercedes 0-916878-06-6)

Printed in the United States of America
10 9 8 7 6

contents

acknowledgments

The Natural Healer's Acupressure Handbook is the product of more than a decade of research in the field of natural health and alternative approaches to conventional Western methods of healing. Along the path, numerous individuals—throughout the world, but especially in southern Florida—have been extremely helpful to its completion, and the author wishes to express his deep appreciation for their assistance. Of these, several deserve special recognition:

Charles P. L. Bestoso—his work has spanned forty years, touched thousands of sufferers, and provided the medical research community a next step.

Ralph Alan Dale, Ed.D., Ph.D., director of the Acupuncture Education Center (Miami)—his efforts have been instrumental in making available the concepts and techniques of the Eastern way of health to both the medical profession and the general public.

Anne Hertz, Lois Wright, Helen Merrill, and Natalie Chapman—whose knowledge and patience have been an invaluable help to the creation of this book.

Barry Sultanoff, M.D.—instructor, friend, and physician in the fullest sense of the word; from his mold, future physicians will be cast.

And Gail Watson, a special friend.

Let me take the first step in introducing you to *The Natural Healer's Acupressure Handbook*. It is my hope that this manual will stimulate your interest in an alternative approach to personal health care. I believe it offers you a new and exciting self-help concept that is fully in keeping with the dynamic changes happening around us.

The decade of the 1960s closed dramatically with man taking a first step onto the moon, probably his greatest technological achievement to date. This ushered in an era of expansion toward seemingly limitless horizons. A new willingness to look within ourselves and to begin a more serious exploration of "innerspace" has been pervasive. As pioneers, seeking guidance on all fronts— from gurus, psychotherapists, and others along the path—we are opening ourselves to multi-cultural influences. The publication of this handbook, with its blending of oriental and occidental viewpoints, attests to the emergence of these trends. Its creation is, in part, a response to the search for alternatives and openness to change that seems to characterize contemporary society.

The handbook emphasizes, as its basic precept, the notion of "first step" in the sense of first aid. Equally important, I feel, is the broader possibility implicit in this "first step" idea: namely that, for some readers, the learning of G-Jo techniques may spark a more general interest in self-sufficiency. Furthermore, the use of these techniques may stimulate an awareness that healing is largely self-generated and that an individual can easily take more initiative in bringing personal health care within his own sphere of influence.

Many centuries ago a significant "first step" was taken by the Greek physician Hippocrates when he embraced, as a basic tenet of healing, the concept of "First, do no harm." Hippocrates understood that the healing process is intrinsic to man, and he was wary of the harm that could be done by misguided interventions into nature's workings. But today, dazzled by our sophisticated knowledge, technology, and treatment approaches, many of us seem to have lost sight of this simple, yet fundamental, principle. Through ignorance—or is it more an *ignore*-ance?—the relevance of this basic principle has been frequently overlooked.

Those of us concerned with personal development recognize health care as an integral part of our evolving consciousness. This "holistic" perspective on the essence of healing presents us with a practical challenge: How can we best utilize the knowledge and services encompassed by Western medicine while maintaining a "healthstyle" attuned to principles of order, balance, and self-reliance? It is to this question that *The Natural Healer's Acupressure Handbook* primarily addresses itself. It thereby provides a viable resource for anyone making the transition to a more self-directed "healthstyle." It presents an alternative way of dealing with many discomforts. Rather than reaching for the medication bottle, one may, with the knowledge gleaned from this handbook (and a minimum of practice) manually stimulate the appropriate point(s). He can thereby take a first, self-initiated step toward promoting symptomatic relief of his discomfort. His decision as to when to consult a physician can then be made more responsibly.

The physician is a valuable resource. He should be sought whenever alternative means of alleviating the problem, including appropriate first-aid or "first-step" techniques, have proven inadequate or when the situation is one that demands his special expertise. A competent physician has many skills that are relevant, useful, and, at times, crucial—for example, the knowledge of how to treat a medical emergency such as diabetic coma or respiratory arrest. The hospital emergency room, however, is not the best setting in which to treat a minor headache, stomach upset, or sleepless night. Yet, the bulk of visits to medical facilities are by clients who lack either the will or the knowledge—often both—to deal responsibly themselves with minor discomforts. It is almost as if the sufferer expects to be met by a white-coated genie, who, with a wave of his magic stethoscope, can banish The Illness from the body. In this abdication of personal power, the individual ultimately reduces himself to a mere spectator, a passive non-participant in his own health care.

The Natural Healer's Acupressure Handbook helps to restore a sense of perspective by detailing a method of self-help, rooted in universal principles of healing, that will "do no harm" if certain clearly stated precautions are followed. It is a method of first aid that is self-contained and can be employed at home or in the woods, without props or other special effects. The author's implicit respect for individual judgment and fostering of self-reliance is something I find particularly refreshing. Here indeed is a guidebook for further ventures along the path of personal responsibility; one can explore it, grow with it, and acquire new skills for his personal "survival kit," thereby laying the ground-work for a sound policy of "health assurance," now and for the future.

Barry Sultanoff, M.D.
Brockport, New York

G-Jo means "first aid"

G-Jo (pronounced "JEE-joh") is roughly translated from the Chinese as meaning "first aid." The techniques described in the following pages, however, are substantially different from the splinting, bandaging, and such one often considers when thinking of Western first aid. The G-Jo techniques primarily rely upon fingertip stimulation of tiny pressure points and are not intended to supersede or replace standard Western first-aid or emergency techniques. Since Western methods are adequately covered in either The American National Red Cross *First Aid Textbook* or the excellent *Emergency Care and Transportation of the Sick and Injured* (please see bibliography), they have not been included here. Instead, this handbook details a number of ancient oriental techniques that may, in certain circumstances, supplement and add to the effectiveness of standard Western first-aid methods.

This traditional, Eastern way of first aid is not limited to emergency situations. The same techniques may be effective in relieving pain or various symptomatic discomforts and provide in the basically healthy person a natural alternative to many non-prescription, over-the-counter pharmaceuticals.

Development of this handbook

This manual of G-Jo techniques grew from a cross-reference file that was developed while teaching and demonstrating the use of various traditional pressure points to groups of medical and non-medical people in southern Florida. Resources included many of the currently available texts dealing with the oriental way of health and healing plus conversations with, and instruction from, masters in the art of acupuncture and the yin/yang theory. Also consulted were a number of professional journals devoted to Eastern and Western medical practice.

In preparing the book, the goal has been to furnish potentially useful, if novel, information in a simple, concise format. The list of symptoms that each point has been historically documented to relieve is not necessarily complete in the following pages. Rather, the included list evolved from recommendations by physicians and outdoorspeople, as well as from personal travel experience in many parts of the world.

Although much of the information presented here has been repeatedly confirmed by personal experience, it has not been possible to gather firsthand knowledge of the efficiency of every point for relieving each symptom ascribed to it. For many symptoms included in this handbook, especially the more serious, Type 2 symptoms, historical documentation has been relied upon. The bibliography at the back of the book lists current titles found especially helpful during the research.

Throughout this book the word "traditional" is used frequently. This refers to those non-Western theories and techniques practiced widely throughout the entire East (Japan, India, etc.) that are based upon the ancient medical and health philosophies of China. These ideas grew from thousands of years of empirical observation and recording. They were first made public some four thousand years ago in what may be the first medical book ever written, *The Yellow Emperor's Classic of Internal Medicine (Huang Ti Nei Ching Su Wen)*, or simply, *The Yellow Emperor's Classic*. It is still a primary text for those interested in the subject of holistic, traditional health and healing.

Paramedical healers and traditional therapies

Every society throughout history has had its healers, medical and non-medical. Sorcerers with secret potions, wise old men and women with vast knowledge of herbs and plants, psychic or spiritually aware individuals—all have played important roles in community health long before formally educated doctors became common. In some societies or subcultures, the non-medical healer still serves a useful purpose and fills a pressing need in treating those people unwilling or unable to seek more conventional medical care.

Today China's health programs—an amalgam of Western and oriental medical practices—are not limited solely to physicians. There are thousands of paramedically trained people who have the responsibility, along with their regular jobs, of acting as a first step in treating neighbors suffering from ill health. In addition, these so-called "barefoot doctors" act to distinguish those sufferers who need only minor care—which the "barefoot doctors" also provide—from the more seriously ill. Patients needing advanced medical treatment are then referred to district or urban hospitals or clinics.

China's non-medical and paramedical programs are probably more advanced than those of any other major country. But in many Western countries, EMT (Emergency Medical Treatment), first-step, and paramedical programs are gaining popularity. There seems little doubt that paramedicine will be one of the most strongly emphasized community health programs for the next several decades. And some of the oriental techniques, especially those rooted in the traditional, holistic philosophy, are well worth considering as adjuncts and complements to standard Western methods.

In addition to external health aids, the body seems to have a complex intuitive system for safeguarding its own health. This often appears as a craving for one food or another (food therapy is one of the most important aspects in the philosophy of traditional healing). We also massage an aching part of our bodies, rub our eyes if they feel tired, or wring our hands when anxious. In so doing, we contact many of the pressure points described in the following pages. At an even less conscious level, the random, daily scratching each of us does in response to an unprovoked itch often stimulates one or more of the body's therapy points while relieving the "purposeless" annoyance.

A brief overview of traditional medical theory

It is traditionally assumed that the body always seeks to heal itself. Traditional therapy—medical, paramedical or non-medical, and first step—serves only one purpose: to change the body's "inner environment" and allow the natural healing process to continue. The sooner these changes are made, the less difficulty the body encounters in continuing the process. In this sense, the use of traditional first-step methods is not thought to "mask" the symptoms or merely to produce analgesia.

Westerners, too, have their own type of first-step therapy, usually in the form of non-prescription, easily available pharmaceuticals, such as aspirin. Many of their beneficial qualities are undeniable, and their uses are manifold. On the other hand, the rise in consumerism has unearthed numerous dangers from abusing chemical compounds that have been mainstays in our existence. Whether or not some over-the-counter pharmaceuticals are potentially dangerous is debatable, but a need certainly exists for a harmless alternative to the *un*healthy aspects of our personal health care programs.

While the thrust of Western (sometimes called *allopathic*) medicine is *curing and healing illness,* traditional medicine is directed more toward *preventing illness.* The traditional physician is first a philosopher, then a doctor. Ideally, his early training has been well grounded in the spiritual aspects of life; then the bulk of his formal education has been devoted to understanding the unified, holistic concept of life (yin/yang theory) and its application to health and healing.

As the Western doctor is taught about germs and viruses, he is trained to see the human body as an entity distinctly separate from its environment—a basically self-contained unit. The traditional doctor, however, sees the body as an integral part of its environment, shaped and controlled by forces that surround and permeate it. That germs and viruses may be present is not denied; instead, they are thought to be responses to a lifestyle that is in disharmony with the immediate environment.

The question of environment is important; it goes far beyond what most Westerners usually take into account. The traditional doctor actually considers two environments: the outer (including weather, home, work surroundings, etc.) and the inner (including the patient's emotions, the existing state of his organs, the strength of his "free will," and the condition of the *bioenergy*—life force—in his body). The skin may be visualized as separating these two environments. If there is harmony on both sides, a person is considered to be in good health. But if there is disharmony and imbalance, poor health, if not already obvious, is imminent.

The nature of one's health is a reflection of the state of the subtle, yet omnipotent, bioenergy the Chinese call *ch'i* (pronounced "chee" or "jee"). Bioenergy is considered to be the essence of life. It surrounds and permeates each of us constantly in a "sea of energy." While not easily explained or defined, the concept of bioenergy is vital to the successful practice of traditional medicine; when bioenergy is understood, the entire traditional way of health and healing makes sound, logical sense.

According to *The Yellow Emperor's Classic*, bioenergy is a universal force, complete in and of itself, which should remain in the normal human body for approximately one hundred years, if one's health is guarded. It is thought to be common to every life form; in fact, some of the same traditional methods used to treat human beings have also been successfully applied to domestic animals for thousands of years.

Bioenergy is thought to have a definite, predictable route through every body—to "flow" along a pathway that traverses the body in a fixed pattern somewhat like the network of a complex railway system. Just as a railway system has important terminals, so there are twelve major organs and organ functions in the body where the bioenergy changes direction along the pathway. It is actually a single, looped circuit; but, for the sake of convenience, the pathway is divided into major routes (meridians) named for the organ or function served by each section of the path. Furthermore, there are numerous interconnections and tiny "stops" along the bioenergy circuit; these "stops" are called *acupoints.*

The nature of bioenergy is to flow smoothly and harmoniously throughout the body. But an infinite number of situations can occur in which the bioenergy may be "warped" out of its synchronized flow. The "warp" can ultimately be traced to a single cause: the body's inner environment is out of balance with its surrounding, outer environment. In other words, environmental imbalance warps the flow of bioenergy. The acupoints along the circuit immediately respond to help readjust the flow; but if the imbalance is not quickly corrected, the warped bioenergy will begin to affect one organ or another. This may lead to increasingly poor health, accompanied, in time, by its overt symptoms (which Western medicine calls "disease"). A specific environmental imbalance creates a specific disease—or rather, dis-*ease*.

Curing an illness, disease, or disorder first requires correcting the environmental imbalance that brought it about, thereby allowing the bioenergy to regain its normal, harmonious flow. The gentle and more preferable way of allowing the body to perform its natural, continuous function of healing is to change slightly the lifestyle back from the state that was offensive. Mild therapeutic exercise (such as *t'ai chi ch'uan*) might be prescribed by the traditional physician in one case, and nontraumatic psychotherapy in another. Food is considered to be medicine and a change of diet is usually included in any therapy.

It is important to note that, in the traditional philosophy, *all* functions of the body—even those thought by Westerners to be "mental" in nature (emotions, for example)—are controlled by the major organs. The body cannot be considered truly healthy without a correspondingly healthy "mind." In fact, mind and body are not regarded as separate units—they are different, yet inseparable expressions of unity and wholeness, and each plays a vital role in the flow of bioenergy. "Good health" means that bioenergy is flowing smoothly to the organs and that they are functioning properly; the mind is peaceful and at one with the body. The person is relaxed, yet alert, and a controlled, positive energy seems to radiate from within.

As previously mentioned, the acupoints apparently respond to any change in the flow of bioenergy. They appear to act somewhat like resistors in an electrical circuit by adjusting the speed and power of the flow. Their response is a kind of fluid elasticity that tightens or slackens as necessary. The effects of this fluctuating tension may even be felt by the preceding or subsequent organ in the flow sequence.

For practical purposes, it may be assumed that the acupoints are directly responsible for the manner in which the bioenergy reaches the organs. By carefully using a number of age-old techniques and theories, the experienced traditional physician can diagnose the nature of any organ malfunction ("too yin" or "too yang") and trace his way back to the "offending" points. The true offense, remember, is an imbalance between the two environments, usually caused by a lifestyle that is contrary to the natural laws governing that specific situation or geographic location.

Once the problem has been diagnosed, the physician might select any number of manipulative techniques for stimulating the acupoints when conditions are too far progressed for the gentler way (food therapy, for example) to be immediately effective. Whatever the method chosen for this artificial, manually-induced adjustment—needles, heat, electricity, or fingertips—it falls into the category of *acupuncture*. Fingertip acupuncture has come to be called "acupressure" in the West.

Some of the acupoints are broad acting and easily found; these are known as *formula* or *cookbook* acupoints. They lend themselves especially well to fingertip stimulation, and because of their broad-acting, pressure-responsive nature, they can be used by nearly anyone upon himself for temporary relief of numerous symptoms. These acupoints are the basis for G-Jo pressure-point stimulation techniques.

A number of Western doctors have recently begun seeking more information about acupuncture techniques and why they work. In an attempt to integrate the underlying traditional philosophies and theories into their own thinking, certain changes have been made. One notable—and questionable—change concerns the concept of bioenergy, a key to the traditional theory. There is no Western equivalent of this presumed vital universal force except for the proverbial and non-scientific "spark of life." Hence, there has been general agreement among many Western doctors practicing acupuncture that the bioenergy, *ch'i,* is actually *nervous* energy—that is, the "electrical" force that travels along the sympathetic and parasympathetic nerve channels.

Contrary to that approach, the traditionalist views bioenergy as being more than just a response to stimuli by the nervous system. And recently, the traditional position appears to have received support from investigative work with advanced electrophotography (Kirlian photography) and non-medical (psychic and spiritual) healers.

Conclusion

For some readers, this handbook will be their only contact with traditional health techniques. For others, it will be a first step in learning more about the fascinating—and ageless—concepts from the East. Either way, it is hoped that the following information will be both beneficial and stimulating enough to the reader to promote a greater sense of self-sufficiency.

In presenting this work, there is no intention to negate the advances made by the Western medical and pharmaceutical industries. On the contrary, any knowledge that adds to the health and welfare of a person can only be considered beneficial, unless abused. The techniques described in the following pages should help the average reader take a more active role in his own health maintenance. By so doing, his pharmacist and physicians are returned to their proper places: vital members of his health team, to be consulted after he has assumed at least a degree of responsibility for his personal well-being.

Finally, the study and practice of the traditional, holistic way of health is more than just an exercise of interesting principles; it is a complete way of life. One can hardly become involved in any facet of human biodynamics without soon realizing the awesome magnitude of forces shaping and controlling each of us. The experience is both enlightening and humbling.

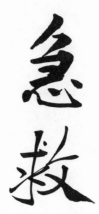

PART I

G-Jo techniques
and how to use them

What is G-Jo?

G-Jo is the translation of the calligraphic characters that mean "first aid" in Chinese. G-Jo (simplified acupressure) is a harmless self-help, fingertip stimulation technique for basically healthy people. Its goal is the temporary reduction or relief of pain or other symptoms of disorders and illness. As soon as symptoms arise, small "points" located near the surface of the skin are briskly stimulated.

This handbook is a catalog of ancient but still widely used therapy pressure points, their locations, and the possible benefits when properly stimulated. Their origin and documentation is, for the most part, oriental; but perhaps as much as three-fourths of the world's population currently uses many of these points in one form or another.

G-Jo is neither a cure nor an alternative to proper medical care. Its use should be limited by the same precautions governing the use of aspirin or other non-prescription, over-the-counter remedies: If pain or symptoms persist, see your doctor immediately.

There are two uses for G-Jo pressure-point stimulation. First, it can be an alternative to non-prescription, over-the-counter remedies for some symptoms; this is called *G-Jo Type 1*. Second, it serves as a possible first-aid or emergency technique, or as a complement to standard Western first-aid or emergency techniques. This is called *G-Jo Type 2* and is intended for one-time or very limited use until you can get medical help. Its use does not replace standard Western first-aid or emergency techniques. The latter are not covered in this handbook, and it is suggested that you also keep a manual of those techniques available.

How to use this handbook

1. Read and understand Part I thoroughly.
2. Check the contents to Part II to find the listing that best describes the symptom or body area to be relieved.
3. Turn to that definition in Part II and see the other suggested symptom definitions, if any. (The abbreviation "etc." that follows many of the additional symptoms or body areas listed in parentheses should be interpreted as a recommendation to refer to the contents for still other relevant possibilities included.)

4. After finding the best symptom definition, note the G-Jo pressure-point numbers(s) listed to the right of the definition.

5. Turn to Part III; refer to the first G-Jo pressure point suggested for relieving the symptom. A cross-reference of symptoms for each point has been added to help you avoid confusion. *The illustration and written instructions are for finding the approximate area only,* since exact pressure points vary slightly between individuals.

6. Find the exact pressure point; then stimulate it deeply and bilaterally (on both sides of the body).

7. If you obtain reduction or relief from the symptom, use no other points. If you obtain *no* reduction or relief from the symptom, try the next suggested point or combination of points. If you still obtain no relief after stimulating each suggested point bilaterally, please see page 9.

How to locate the exact G-Jo pressure point

There are two measurements you should know to find the approximate location of your G-Jo points.

1. *The width of one hand:* This refers to the distance across the rear-most knuckles (see illustration A).

2. *The width of one thumb:* This refers to the distance across the widest part of the thumb, generally just below the nail (see illustration B).

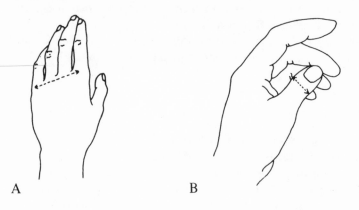

A   B

One or both of these measurements are used from easily found "landmarks" on your body to find the approximate location of each G-Jo pressure point.

For example, G-Jo point number 9 is found the width of one hand below the bottom of the kneecap, then the width of one thumb toward the outside of the leg (in the direction of the small toe). First, place your left hand just below the bottom of your right kneecap and make a mental note of the lowest point your hand reaches (see illustrations C and D). Then, from the center of that spot, measure outward the width of your left thumb (see illustrations E and F). Where the farthest side of your thumb lies is the beginning area to probe; G-Jo point number 9 will be found near that location. Reverse the process to find the same G-Jo point on your left leg.

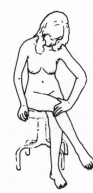

C

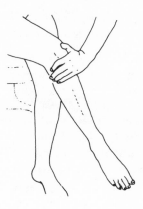

D

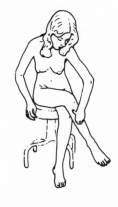

E

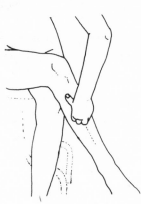

F

If you want to find a G-Jo point on another person, you must remember to use *his* hand and thumb to measure on *his* body. Your hand may be too large—say, for a small child—or too small for accurate measuring.

Next, to locate the exact spot, begin *deeply* probing the area on your body that most closely corresponds to the illustration *until you feel a distinct twinge of sensitivity*. That is the exact pressure point. Probe deeply enough to make you wince.

Use the *tip* of your finger or thumb—not the pad or fleshy part, because the surface is too broad to find the tiny pressure point—until the point announces itself with the "loud" twinge of sensitivity. While the entire area may at first seem pressure-sensitive, with a little practice you will soon be able to separate the exact point from the near-point.

If the point does not announce itself clearly, you may need to apply more pressure. Some points are not easily found. Finding the best point if several possibilities are listed is a trial-and-error process; however, that point is often distinctly more pressure-sensitive than other recommended points.

How to stimulate the G-Jo pressure point

After finding the most pressure-sensitive spot, stimulate *deeply* (with about 20 pounds of pressure) and briskly, generally in a counterclockwise direction, on both sides of the body. The fingertip—again, not the pad or fleshy part—and the skin should move together during the stimulation; the fingertip should *not* just rub over the surface of the skin. Stimulate for 15 to 20 seconds; then stimulate the bilateral point identically. It is important to keep at least the left- and right-hand working fingernails clipped short.

Sometimes more pressure is needed than you can exert using your fingertip. In that case, use your knuckle, thumb, or even a utensil such as the blunt end of a felt-tipped marker.

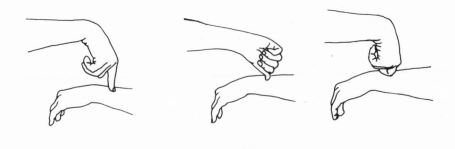

This . . .   this . . .   this . . .

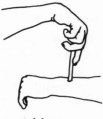
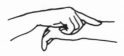

or this . . .   *but not this!*

It is difficult to apply too much pressure; however, it is quite easy not to apply enough pressure. Properly done, there will often be a "memory" remaining at the stimulation site for a few minutes. Bruising usually means that the G-Jo stimulation was too deep, though for some people who bruise easily, even a small amount of pressure will leave a discoloration.

Fear of inflicting pain on yourself may initially magnify your sensitivity or lower your "pain threshold." But after stimulating G-Jo points a few times, this fear is usually overcome. If you continue to find it difficult to stimulate the G-Jo pressure point deeply enough, perhaps a friend or member of your family would do it for you.

Do not overstimulate a point. Stop when you obtain relief, and do *not* use other numbered points to reinforce the effect. Stimulate only when symptoms arise and try to be as relaxed as possible. When relief is obtained, do not immediately "test" the injured or afflicted area, as this may reestablish the bioenergy imbalance. Instead, relax a bit, then *gently* begin using the afflicted area.

As previously mentioned, with the exception of those G-Jo pressure points lying atop the spine or the front mid-line (frontal meridian), each G-Jo point is duplicated on either side of your body. The selected point should be identically stimulated bilaterally (same pressure, same amount of time) before stimulating a new point. It doesn't matter if you first stimulate the right side or the left, as long as you immediately duplicate the stimulation on the other side. (Later, with more practice, you may find one side is more effective for relieving some symptoms and less effective for others.)

Rarely, a symptom might call for the stimulation of a second or even a third point. In that case, the same rules should be followed: Stimulate the first suggested point bilaterally, then the next. The order of their stimulation is unimportant except when specifically noted in the text.

Precisely how stimulation causes relief is not completely understood, but it helps if you will think of your body as a self-sustaining machine that works automatically. It has a number of "dials," however, which allow the operator (you) manually to override and slightly adjust some of its functions temporarily. When you stimulate a G-Jo pressure point, you are, in effect, "turning a dial." The vital bioenergy you are adjusting has an effect upon a servomechanism (organ); this in turn, may affect the malfunction (symptom) that you hope to relieve.

According to traditional oriental theory, your machine (body) has a limited functional capacity (life-span) and begins self-destructing near its natural end. Its capacity may be briefly prolonged (with medicine and medical equipment) or dramatically shortened (say, by an accident). But poor maintenance—that is, improper diet, unhealthy mental attitudes, irregular activity and exercise—gradually changes the bioenergy flow and balance until premature erosion (illness) and malfunction occur. At that state, your body/machine demands a tune-up; usually it also requires important changes in healthstyle. (For further information about the concepts of traditional oriental health and medical techniques, please refer to the introduction.)

The chain of events following successful G-Jo stimulation

If the pressure-point stimulation is effective, the following might ideally occur:

1. Immediate reduction or relief of the symptom, often followed by a further, gradual easing of discomfort.

2. A release of tension, sometimes throughout your entire body, of which you might not previously have been aware, often accompanied by light perspiration, release of gas, or other responses. These responses are called "acupressure reactions."

3. Later, the symptom might return, but not as strongly as before. The point you first stimulated that best relieved the symptom should again be stimulated.

4. The timespan between necessary stimulations should lengthen until, after three or four restimulations, G-Jo techniques are no longer necessary.

Such a chain of events might be especially true when relieving minor symptoms as soon as they are first noticed. The more serious or chronic the problem, the less effective G-Jo pressure-point stimulation may be, and the more important it is to get immediate medical help.

What to do if G-Jo techniques fail to relieve symptoms

If you get no relief after trying each suggested point for a symptom, it may be due to one or more of the following causes:
1. You may have made the wrong analysis of the problem (and used the wrong point). Try redefining what you hope to relieve. It is often possible to define your problem in three ways: first, *cause* (for instance, seasickness); second, *effect* (in this case, nausea); and third, *affected body area* (stomach, head, etc.).
2. You may not have stimulated a point, but rather an area near the point. Make sure the point announced itself with a strong twinge of sensitivity when stimulated.
3. You may have stimulated the proper point, but not briskly or deeply enough. Review instructions.
4. You may have stimulated the proper point, but under conditions when G-Jo stimulation should not have been used. Review these conditions listed below.

When not to use G-Jo pressure-point stimulation

Except under conditions requiring first aid or emergency care, when its use should be very limited, you should *not* consider G-Jo pressure-point stimulation in the following situations:
1. As a treatment for a chronic, long-standing illness, problem, or disorder.
2. Within four hours of taking *any* drugs (including aspirin), medications, intoxicating drinks or food, or medicinal herbs.
3. If you take regular, daily medications (except vitamins).
4. If you have a known heart condition or suffer from a disorder involving tissue change or degeneration such as serious arthritis, cancer or cancerous growths, cataracts, tumors, varicose veins, etc.
5. Immediately before or within half an hour after bathing in hot water, eating a heavy meal, or doing strenuous physical activity.
6. If you are temporarily in an agitated emotional state, such as rage, avoid Type 1 use until composure has been regained.
7. If the suggested point lies beneath a scar, wart, mole, varicose vein, swollen or inflamed skin, etc.
8. If you are pregnant, especially after the third month.
9. If you are a woman and the suggested pressure point lies upon the breast.

In these circumstances, the use of any traditional oriental manipulative technique—not only G-Jo pressure-point stimulation—is customarily restricted to physicians, if used at all. The bioenergy is assumed to be too imbalanced then for the untrained person to deal with effectively.

One final caution: If you find G-Jo stimulation temporarily relieves your symptom, but the symptom keeps recurring with equal frequency and severity, you should consult your doctor.

Using G-Jo pressure-point stimulation on others

The G-Jo principles and pressure points are based on natural laws governing every human body, so it is possible to use the described techniques on someone other than yourself. G-Jo pressure-point stimulation, however, is a form of massage. Since most states have laws prohibiting the performance of remedial massage by unlicensed people, you should limit G-Jo pressure-point stimulation to yourself, or, if necessary, to members of your family.

When used upon others, there are additional steps to be taken:
1. Explain to the person what you are going to do; tell him that you are looking for the most pressure-sensitive point, and that when you find it and stimulate it there should be some discomfort.
2. Get verbal—or at least facial—feedback during the stimulation. "Is this the point?" or "How does this feel?" should be asked repeatedly, since he will often have an intuitive feeling that the point should be slightly more in one direction or another, or that one point is useful while another is not.

It is also important to remember that working with another is a team effort, not a superior/inferior relationship; you are providing the knowledge and the necessary pressure while it is his body that is relieving the symptom, if the G-Jo stimulation is successful.

"Control centers"

While each G-Jo pressure point might be considered a control center, some points have long histories of effectiveness in temporary relief of definite, but poorly understood, physical reactions. Often these reactions are in response to emotionally charged situations (fear control centers, temper control centers, etc.); or to natural or physical excesses (sweating control centers, warm-up control centers, etc.); or to underlying health problems (fever control centers, etc.). The points for control centers are intended for strictly limited use.

The reason these control centers may be helpful, according to traditional oriental theory, is that all responses and reactions are linked to one organ or another, and stimulating a G-Jo pressure-point control center is thought to trigger a balancing response in the affected organ or organs.

Some additional advice

1.   In stimulating G-Jo pressure points, a feeling of relaxed openness is better than doubtful skepticism, while a positive, confident attitude is better still. Practice adds to this sense of confidence. According to traditional theory, though, the results of stimulating pressure points are mechanical rather than mystical; and properly stimulating the best point for a particular symptom should relieve it as well for the skeptic as for the "believer." After a few symptoms have been successfully relieved with G-Jo pressure-point stimulation, skepticism and lack of confidence are usually overcome.

2.   It is helpful to memorize some of the information contained in this section. Besides remembering the conditions under which G-Jo stimulation should not be used, you should also memorize the G-Jo pressure points marked with a double asterisk (**), as well as their important uses. These points are the most broad acting and most commonly used. They include numbers 4, 5, 7, 9, 10, and 13. Points of slightly lesser importance are marked with a single asterisk (*). These might be memorized as well, but only as an added convenience.

3.   Remember, G-Jo pressure-point stimulation will not interfere with any benefits resulting from Western first-aid, paramedical, or medical techniques. A holistic approach to health encourages the use of all relevant techniques with the ultimate goal being a natural lifestyle in which drugs and chemical medications are used only after drugless therapy has failed. However, as previously noted, G-Jo pressure-point stimulation should not be employed within four hours after taking any drugs or medications; nor should it be considered an alternative, except in emergency, if you take regular, prescribed medications.

Summary

1. G-Jo pressure-point stimulation is not an alternative to proper medical care; its goal is the temporary reduction or relief of pain and symptoms of many disorders and illnesses.
2. Under some circumstances, G-Jo pressure-point stimulation might be considered as an alternative to aspirin or other non-prescription medications; or it might be used on a strictly limited basis to complement standard Western first-aid or emergency techniques.
3. After finding the page illustrating the point with which you hope to relieve your symptom, read the description of its location and *deeply* probe the approximate area for the most pressure-sensitive spot; this is the G-Jo pressure point.
4. The G-Jo pressure point should be stimulated *deeply* with the finger*tip* (finger and skin moving together, not the finger rubbing over the skin) for 15 or 20 seconds in a brisk, generally counter-clockwise direction. Stimulation should be done bilaterally with about 20 pounds of pressure.
5. Stop when you obtain relief or reduction of the symptom; do not overstimulate the same or other points in an effort to reinforce the action. Do not strenuously test the relieved body area.
6. If you obtain no relief or reduction of the symptom, refer to page 9.
7. Stimulate the G-Jo pressure point only when symptoms arise; begin stimulation as soon as possible after the symptom arises.
8. G-Jo pressure-point stimulation is for basically healthy people except under emergency circumstances. Please memorize the list of conditions under which G-Jo stimulation should *not* be used.
9. The G-Jo pressure points marked with a double asterisk (**) are the most commonly used and should be memorized. Of slightly lesser importance, those points with a single asterisk (*) might also be memorized.
10. Symptoms are often associated with underlying health problems; if the symptom you are trying to relieve persists, see your doctor.

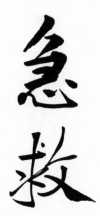

PART II

**symptoms, body areas,
and control centers**

contents

Carbon monoxide poisoning
Cataracts
Cauterization
"Charley horse"
Chemical burns
Chest
Child birth
Choking
Cholera
Claustrophobia
Coccyx
Cold (body too cold)
Colds and influenza
Colitis
Collapse
Concussion
Congestion, sinus or nasal
Conjunctivitis (pink eye)
Constipation (costiveness)
Convulsions
Convulsions in children
Cough
Cramps, menstrual
Cramps and spasms, muscular
Cuts
Cystitis
Deafness (sudden, acute)
Dehydration
Dental work
Diabetes (diabetes mellitus)
Diarrhea
Dislocation of bones
Dizziness
Drowning
Drowsiness
Drug Abuses
Dysentery
Dyspepsia
Dyspnea
Ear
Eczema
Edema
Elbow (including "tennis elbow")
Electric shock(electrocution)

Energy
Epilepsy and epileptic seizures
Exhaustion, physical and/or mental,
Exposure
Eye
Face
Fainting (syncope)
Fatigue
Fear control centers
Fear in children
Fever control centers
Fingers
Fits
Flatulence
Flu
Food poisoning
Foot
Forearm
Fracture
Frostbite
Gall bladder
Gas, intestinal and/or stomach
Gastrointestinal system
Genital weakness, pain, etc.
Genitourinary system
Gingivitis
Goiter
Gonorrhea
Gout
Gunshot wounds
Hand
Hangover
Hay fever
Head
Headaches
Heart
Heart attack, heart failure
Heartburn
Heat (body too hot)
Heat rash (miliaria, "prickly heat ")
Hemorrhage (bleeding)
Hemorrhoids (piles)
Hepatitis

16

Hernia (rupture)
Herpes simplex virus
Hiccough (hiccups)
High blood pressure
Hip
Hives and rash (urticaria)
Hunger control centers
Hypertension (high blood pressure)
Hyperventilation
Hypoglycemia
Hypotension (low blood pressure)
Hysteria
Impetigo and eczema
Indigestion
Infection
Influenza
Injuries
Insanity
Insect bites and stings
Insensibility
Insomnia
Insulin reactions
Intestinal problems
Intoxication
Jaundice
Jaw, lower
Kidneys
Knee
Laryngitis
Leg
Lethargy
Lightheadedness
Lips
Liver
Lockjaw
Low blood pressure
Low blood sugar
Lumbago
Lungs
Malaria
Man-o-war burns
Measles
Memory control centers
Meningitis

Menstruation
Mental disturbances
Migraine
Miliaria
Mosquito bites
Motion sickness
Mountain sickness (hypoxia)
Mouth
Mumps
Muscles
Nasal congestion (catarrh)
Nausea
Neck
Nervousness
Neuralgia
Night sweating
Nightmares
Nosebleed (epistaxis)
Numbness
Ovaries
Overheating (body too hot)
Pain control centers
Pancreas
Panic
Paralysis
Paralysis, infantile
Peritonitis
Pleurisy
Pneumonia
Posion ivy, oak or sumac
Poisoning by mouth (oral poison-
    ing)
Poisoning, carbon monoxide
Poisoning, food
Poisoning, ptomaine
"Possession by devils "
Prostate
Puncture wounds
Queasiness
Rabies
Rash
Rectum
Respiratory system
Restlessness

Retching
Rheumatism
Rhinitis
Scalds
Sciatica
Scorpion stings
Seasickness
Sedation and tranquilization control centers
Sexual organs
Shingles
Shock
Shock, electric
Shock, emotional
Shoulder
Sinusitis
Skin
Sleep control centers
Sluggishness
Small intestines
Smoke inhalation
Smoking control centers
Snakebite
Sneezing control centers
Sore throat
Spasm, muscular
Spider bites
Spleen and pancreas
Sprains, muscular
Stage fright
Stamina control centers
Stimulation
Stings, bee and wasp
Stings, scorpion
Stomach
Strains, muscular
Strength, loss of, or to regain
Stricture of urine
Stroke
Stuttering control center

Styes
Suffocation
Suicidal tendencies
Sunburn
Sunstroke
Sweating control centers
Syncope
Tachycardia, paroxysmal
Temper control centers
Tennis elbow
Testicles, including crushed testicles
Tetanus (lockjaw)
Thigh
Thirst control centers
Throat
Toes
Tongue
Tonsilitis
Toothache
Tooth extraction, drilling, etc.
Torticollis (stiff neck)
Travel sickness
Tumors
Ulcers, intestinal
Ulcers, peptic
Unconsciousness, causes unknown
Urinary control centers
Urticaria
Varicose veins
Venereal disease
Vertigo
Vomiting and retching
Warm-up control centers
Wasp stings
Weakness, physical
Whiplash (neck injury)
Wounds
Wrist
Yawning control center

Abdomen, lower (also see: Appendicitis; Peritonitis; etc.): the area between the navel and the pubic region. Sharp pain in the right side could indicate appendicitis.

3	
7	
9	
10	
14	
36	
50	violent pain
68	
73	abdomen distended

Abdomen, upper (also see: Stomach; etc.): the area between the chest and the navel.

7	
9	
36	
95	

Acne (also see: Allergies, non-specific; Skin; etc.): eruptions on the face, chest, back, etc.

2	
13	
27	
28	
81	esp. upper back, shoulders
84	

Allergies, non-specific (also see: Sneezing control centers; other symptoms associated with allergies): a repeated bodily reaction upon

2	
11	sneezing
27	
28	

exposure to an allergenic substance such as food, feathers, etc.

80B	hay fever-like allergy
112	
115	sneezing

Altitude sickness: see Mountain sickness (hypoxia).

Amnesia: see Apoplexy (stroke); Memory control centers; etc.: an organic and/or emotionally induced partial or total loss of recall or memory.

Anger: see Temper control centers.

Angina pectoris (also see: Chest; Heart; Heart attack, heart failure; Pain; etc.): deep spasmodic pain often radiating to the left arm and shoulder. It is often triggered by an emotional or physically taxing experience. *Get medical help immediately.*

10
15

Ankle: see Foot.

Anxiety (also see: Fear control centers; Hysteria; etc.): warranted or unwarranted fear of a future event or condition.

4	
10	
15	especially stage fright
16	
41	
45	
69	
71	with palpitations
82	

Apoplexy (stroke): the result of a blood clot or hemorrhage to the brain or a major organ. Its symptoms are varied depending upon the degree of damage. There may be unconsciousness, heavy breathing and/or paralysis of either or both the upper or lower half of one side of the sufferer's body. When there is unconsciousness, the pupils of the eyes may be unevenly dilated. If there is heavy breathing and unconsciousness, there is the possibility of the sufferer choking from his own saliva. Turn him on his side to allow the saliva

10	
19	
20	left side only, followed in ten minutes by 21

to drool from his mouth. *Get medical help immediately.*

Appendicitis (also see: Abdomen, lower; etc.): an inflammation of the appendix, located below and slightly to the right of the navel. Its symptoms include severe pain and tenderness in the right-hand side of the lower abdomen, vomiting, nausea, diarrhea, and generally a sickly appearance. This may be a serious problem; there is the possibility of the appendix rupturing. *Get medical help immediately.*

14
83
91

Arm (also see: Elbow; Forearm; Hand; Shoulder): including both the arm and the armpit.

2
4
10   armpit painful and swollen
18   armpit painful and swollen
21
29
39
44   pain in upper arm
61
88
103
116

Arteriosclerosis: no G-Jo pressure-point stimulation to be used.

Arthritis, chronic: no G-Jo pressure-point stimulation to be used.

Asphyxia (suffocation — also see: Choking; Drowning; etc.): unconsciousness resulting from too much carbon dioxide (CO_2) in the blood. An emergency/death-pending condition; G-Jo pressure-point stimulation does not replace standard Western first-aid or emergency techniques. *Get medical help immediately.*

8
17   if face is blue
18   if face is pale
48
58

Asthma and asthmatic breathing, wheezing, etc. (also see: Asphyxia; Dyspnea; Hysteria; etc.): massive narrowing and constriction of the air passages in the throat. Its symptoms include coughing, wheezing, panic, etc. *Get medical help immediately.*

1	
11	
13	
18	
61	
81	
84	
85	
87	

Athlete's foot (also see: Foot): A damp, itching rot between the toes.

92

Back, lower and/or upper (also see: Lumbago; Pain; Sciatica; etc.).

3 plus 5	
5	lower back
7	lower back
9	lower back
13	middle back
29	upper back
38	
47	
51	
58	lower back
61	
69	lower back
70	lower back
80B	
83	upper back
103	upper back
114	
116	upper back

Bee Stings: see Stings, bee and wasp.

Beriberi: a problem caused by a lack of vitamin B_1 (thiamine). Uncommon in most industrialized parts of the world, its symptoms include disturbed sleep, irritability, lack of concentration, poor memory, and abdominal disorders.

35
91

Bioenergy control centers (also see: Stamina control centers; etc.): Bioenergy is the life energy (*ch'i* in Chinese) that all traditional oriental therapy seeks to balance. Chronic excesses or deficiencies of bioenergy require changes in diet, lifestyle, exercise activity, and/or medication. *Gentle* stimulation may be

6
8
9
26
31
32
47
69
97

temporarily helpful if you want "more energy"; *brisk* stimulation may be temporarily helpful if you are feeling "too energetic."

Birth, giving: see Childbirth.

Bites, animal, human and insect (also see: Snakebite; Stings, bee and wasp; Stings, scorpion; etc.): If you are bitten by a wild creature, there is a possibility of rabies, especially if the bite is from a skunk, squirrel, raccoon or other small mammal. Try capturing the animal alive for observation in captivity. Killing the animal is less desirable; but if done, keep the head refrigerated until it can be tested in a laboratory.

20	
22	including tetanus
24	
32	especially rabid animal bite
61	tetanus prevention

Bites, spider (also see: Stings, bee and wasp; Stings, scorpion; etc.): Many spiders are somewhat poisonous, but the two most common truly poisonous spiders are the (female) Black Widow and the Brown Household (or Brown Recluse).

The Black Widow is found throughout the Americas and is shiny black, about the size of a thumbnail, with an orange-to-red hourglass design on her "stomach." Often found outdoors, (especially in old, rotted wood areas), nearly two-thirds of all Black Widow bites are suffered by men, on or about the genital region, from using wooden outhouse seats.

Conversely, women usually suffer bites of the Brown Recluse, which is generally found indoors in dark areas such as clothes closets.

Symptoms include pain, abdominal cramps, sometimes paralysis, and tenderness, redness, and swelling around the bitten area. *Get medical help immediately.*

20	right foot only, when skin is red, swollen, waxy-looking
22	skin is cold
24	skin is hot, red, inflamed
25	

Bladder (also see: Cystitis; Genitourinary system; Urine control centers): the organ of accumulation for urine.

bladder	
3	54
9	56
24	62
25	75
28	114

Bleeding, arterial (also see: Bleeding, venous; Hemorrhage; etc.): bright red blood being pumped from a wound in a throbbing, pulsing manner. This may be an emergency/death-pending condition.

110	left side only
111	anywhere in body

Place a cloth or rag over the wound and press down tightly. While holding it in place, apply deep pressure into the area where the chest joins the left armpit and hold the pressure (illustrated point no. 110). Or place your right fist in your left armpit and clamp your left arm down onto the fist, holding it tightly. The point is found on the *chest* side of the armpit, rather than on the *arm* side.

G-Jo pressure-point stimulation does not replace standard Western emergency or first-aid techniques. *Get medical help immediately.*

Bleeding, venous: (also see: Bleeding, arterial; Hemorrhage, etc.): dark, purplish blood flowing (rather than spurting) from a wound. This may be an emergency/death-pending condition. Follow the instruction for Bleeding, arterial, except use the *right* armpit, rather than the left. *Get medical help immediately.*

110	right side only
111	anywhere in body

Bleeding in general: see Hemorrhage; Nosebleed (epistaxis); etc.

Bleeding gums: see Gingivitis.

Blisters (also see affected areas such as Hand, etc.): watery, raised areas just below the surface of the skin. Caused either by friction or pinching (blood blisters), you should avoid breaking the blisters, if possible.

2	
13	pain
27	
28	

Boils, styes, carbuncles (also see: Skin; etc.): localized "staph" infections of varying degrees of severity. They are often found

1	styes
2	
27	

around the eyes (styes), neck, back, or buttocks.

28	
29	boils
35	carbuncles

Bones: This point is used regularly to help
fractured bones knit quickly and well.

42

Brain: see Concussion; Meningitis; etc.

Breasts: *Any lump or swelling in the breast
should receive prompt medical attention.*

10
29
97

Breath control centers (also see: Bioenergy
control centers; Stamina control centers;
etc.): may temporarily help ease panting and
breathlessness from exertion, etc. Stimulating
these points may also be helpful in preparing
for a situation when heavy breathing is
anticipated.

20	breathlessness and pant-ing
45	
65	
105	to prepare for a situa-tion requiring heavy breathing

Breathing, difficult and labored: see Dyspnea.

Bronchitis (also see: Chest; Cough; Respiratory system; Throat; etc.): an inflammation
of the bronchial "tree" whose symptoms
include: fever, pains in the back and muscles,
headache, etc.

1
11
44
53
55
78
86
96
97
112

Bruises (also see: Wounds, etc.): discoloration
and/or injury beneath the skin resulting from
wounds when blood vessels have been ruptured.

21	if skin is not broken
26	if skin is broken
103	

Burns and scalds, including sunburn: There
are different types of burns as well as degrees
of severity:
    a. Thermal (heat) burns: Immerse the area
    in a slush of freshwater ice and water, or
    cover the burned area with a grated potato;

2	
5	pain
24	especially sunburn
27	
28	
75	

b. Chemical burns: Flush chemicals from the tissue immediately;

c. Sunburn (also see: Sunstroke): Covering the burned area with vinegar or aloe gel may be helpful.

For more serious burns, drink plenty of water with a little salt and baking soda added to help replace the salty fluids of the body and reduce the possibility of shock. Do not apply ointments or pastes such as baking soda in the case of a severe burn; they will only have to be scraped off at a hospital or burn center. *Get medical help immediately.*

Bursitis (also see affected areas, such as Shoulder, etc.): an inflammation between moving joints.

11
37

Buttocks (also see: Hip; etc.).

50
63

Cancer and cancerous growths: No G-Jo pressure-point stimulation to be used.

Cardiac arrest (also see: Heart attack, heart failure; etc.): Make sure the victim is not *choking.* Cardiac arrest is an emergency condition where the heart stops pumping (contracting) or slows so that an inadequate supply of blood moves through the blood vessels. Its symptoms include sudden unconsciousness, very faint or no pulse, absence of heartbeat, absence of breathing. G-Jo pressure-point stimulation does not replace standard Western emergency or first-aid techniques. *Get medical help immediately.* Note the exact time the cardiac arrest took place. This will be very helpful for a doctor or EMT personnel.

8
76   squeeze and pump
         briefly, then see:
         Heart attack, heart
         failure

Car sickness: see Seasickness; Travel sickness; etc.

Carbon monoxide poisoning: see Poisoning, carbon monoxide.

Cataracts: no G-Jo pressure-point stimulation to be used.

Cauterization: strictly an emergency survival technique to stop severe bleeding. Heat a knife over an open fire until the blade is red hot; this both sterilizes it and makes it a cauterizing tool. Then touch the heated metal to the open wound, scorching the flesh until the wound is sealed.

If cauterizing yourself, first lie down and think about where the knife would fall since fainting is possible.

"Charley horse": see Strains, muscular.

Chemical burns: see Burns and scalds.

Chest (also see: Lungs; Respiratory system; etc.).

1
4
10
13

Childbirth: No G-Jo pressure-point stimulation to be used except in emergency situations, after the birth has begun, to help ease a difficult delivery. G-Jo pressure-point stimulation does not replace standard Western first-aid or emergency techniques. *Get medical help immediately.*

5
7
13
75   to ease delivery
94

Choking: Symptoms of mild choking include gagging and coughing or other indications of partial stoppage of air. Severe choking may be an emergency/death-pending condition; the foreign object may either be lodged in the throat or the lungs.

If choking is mild, allow the victim to clear

8
12   after the object has
        been removed from
        the victim's throat
88   object stuck in throat

his own air passages by coughing; do not try talking to him. If choking becomes severe, do the following:

a. **An infant choking** — hold him upside down by his ankles, open his mouth and pull out his tongue. Shake him, if necessary, and let the swallowed object fall to the floor. If the object does not fall to the floor and the infant can breathe, it probably means the object has descended into his lungs. *Get medical help immediately;*

b. **An older child choking** — hoist him over a chair or your arm or leg so that his head hangs lower than his chest. Strike him sharply between the shoulder blades *once*, open his mouth and pull out his tongue. Clear his throat with your fingers;

c. **An adult choking** — follow the same instructions for an older child, being sure that his head is lower than his neck. Or do a "bear hug" after first attempting to clear his air passage with your fingers. Stand behind the victim with both your arms around his waist; make a fist and place your other hand over it so that you are holding the victim with your hands just below the bottom of his rib cage. Apply a sharp, upward thrusting pressure; this will force the always present residual air in the lungs out and should clear the air passage with an audible "pop."

"Cafe coronary" (choking while eating) is not uncommon, especially with older adults who have been drinking before dinner, and its symptoms resemble a heart attack. If the victim cannot talk, or shakes his head "no" when you ask him if he can talk, he is choking.

After removing the object, *get medical help immediately*, especially if the victim was without air for more than a minute or the object seemed to be in his lungs. G-Jo pressure-point stimulation does not replace standard Western first-aid or emergency techniques.

Cholera (also see: Cramps, muscular; Diarrhea; Dysentery; etc.): a disease from contaminated food or water which may become epidemic. Its symptoms include severe diarrhea, vomiting, muscular cramps and spasms, dehydration, drying up of urine (oliguria), and collapse. The disease is common in many Asiatic countries and usually runs its course within two weeks. Cholera is an extremely serious problem, but it is immunizable. *Get medical help immediately.*

2
4
6
9   use with all points
17
23
44
61
88
95

Claustrophobia (including Claustrophilia—also see: Anxiety; Hysteria; Nervousness; etc.): an abnormal fear (claustrophobia) or desire (claustrophilia) to be in a small, tightly enclosed space.

18

Coccyx: the small, bony protrusion at the bottom of the spine, commonly called the "tailbone".

19

Cold (When you are too cold or chilled): see Warm-up control centers.

Colds and influenza (also see accompanying symptoms such as: Cough; Headache; Nasal congestion; etc.): The word "colds" has been applied to many symptoms that come together and last for about seven days; an upper respiratory infection.

Symptoms of colds and influenza include fever, cough, dull aches and pains, nasal congestion (catarrh), etc. At the first sign of these symptoms, also wrap a cube of ice to the bottom of each big toe with strips of rag.

1
2
4
9
13
23
69
81
89
98
112
also place ice cube on pad of each big toe

29

Let the ice stay for about twenty minutes; do this several times a day, or as necessary. The ice acts to "brake the flow of bioenergy" past an important cold and influenza control center according to traditional theory.

Colitis (also see: Abdomen, lower; Gastrointestinal system, etc.): a usually chronic inflammation of the colon.

1
7
9
24

Collapse: see Exhaustion; Mental disturbances; Shock; etc.: severe depression or exhaustion brought about by physical and/or mental problems. *Get medical help immediately.*

Concussion (also see: Hemorrhage; Shock; Unconsciousness; etc.): the state resulting from being violently struck or shaken about the head and/or the spine. Its symptoms include headache, unconsciousness, heavy, slow pulse (but not always), reddish-purple face (again, not always), heavy breathing, and, if the skull is broken, there may be blood in the ear canal and bleeding from the nose or mouth. Later, especially in the case of an injured brain, there may be a weak and rapid pulse, ashen-colored face or the breathing may be labored.

Concussion is an emergency condition. The victim should lie extremely quiet; if his face is reddish-purple, his head should be elevated. If his face is ashen and pale, his feet should be elevated. *Get medical help immediately.* Symptoms of concussion may not present themselves for some time after the incident.

1
8
13
18
19
20 left side only, followed
     in ten minutes by
21 if blood is oozing from
     ears, nose, or mouth
26 if injury is at the spine

Congestion, sinus or nasal: see Nasal congestion (catarrh).

Conjunctivitis (pink eye—also see: Eye): an inflammation and reddening of the membrane (conjunctiva) covering the front of the eye.

1
13
18
50
80A

Constipation (costiveness — also see: Gastro-intestinal system): a condition where the bowels move infrequently or with great difficulty. It may be chronic or acute and is associated with a great number of physical or mental disturbances.

6
7
8
9
34
48
62
65
67
68
71
95

Convulsions (also see: Convulsions in children; Epilepsy and epileptic seizures; etc.): general, involuntary muscular spasms that may be of a dramatic and violent nature and which usually occur in an unconscious state.

G-Jo pressure-point stimulation does not replace standard Western first-aid or emergency techniques. The most important consideration is to help the sufferer avoid hurting himself. *Get medical help immediately.*

5
12   face is bright red; eyes dry
32   epileptic seizure
33   violent intestinal convulsions and spasms; eyes wet
34   hysterical convulsions; face is pale
35
70
99

Convulsions in children (also see: Convulsions; Epilepsy and epileptic seizures; etc.): Convulsions in children are not uncommon. High fever is one of the most common triggering agents for convulsions in children. In some cases, children feign or imitate convulsions for attention-getting purposes, especially if they have convulsed earlier in their lives. Besides the suggested points, also massage the convulsing child's earlobes. *Get medical help immediately.*

5
35
70
99

Cough (also see: Bronchitis; Colds and influenza; etc.): This condition may arise from a

1
4

number of causes and be symptomatic of many ailments.

9
10
11
18
20
23   hacking cough
44
48
55
61
64
65
81
97
107

Cramps, menstrual: see Menstruation

Cramps and spasms, muscular (also see: Pain; etc.): painful, involuntary spasms of muscles anywhere in the body.

17
35
57
62
65
115

Cuts: see Wounds; specific portions of the body that are affected, such as Hand, etc.

Cystitis (also see: Bladder; Genitourinary system; etc.): an inflammation of the bladder. Often there is a need to urinate, but only a few drops are passed, generally accompanied by a cutting, burning sensation.

6
7
19
24
41
65
70

Deafness (sudden, acute — also see: Ear): total or partial loss of hearing, often associated with inflammation or growths within the ear canal, but may stem from a number of causes. *Get medical help immediately.*

56
64
89
98
99
100
106

Dehydration: see Shock; Thirst control centers; etc.: a potentially dangerous state where the body tissues contain insufficient fluids. *Get medical help immediately.*

Dental work (also see: Toothache; Toothache, upper jaw; etc.): The G-Jo pressure-points may be helpful for those who cannot have or choose not to have anaesthesia for dental work.

15	before dental work begins
16	before dental work begins
26	every two hours after dental work is finished, until pain and symptoms subside
56	during dental work

Diabetes (diabetes mellitus — also see: Spleen and pancreas; etc.): a complex disease resulting from the underproduction of insulin, a vital chemical in the body's handling of sugar. A diabetic sufferer needs an addition of insulin to compensate for its lack within his body. Without it, he may gradually or rapidly slip into a state of unconsciousness. Symptoms of insufficient insulin include fever, dry mouth, intense thirst, and the smell of nail polish remover (acetone) on his breath. He may appear to be very ill with flushed, dry skin. Vomiting and abdominal pain may be present; he may be hungry for air, but not for food, and his vision may be dim. This is an emergency condition; *get medical help immediately*. G-Jo pressure-point stimulation does not replace insulin or proper medical attention.

6
7
9
11
19
20
28
72
79
109

Diarrhea (loose, runny bowels — also see: Dysentery; Gastrointestinal system; etc.): this condition may be symptomatic of any number of minor or major problems. If the condition continues for more than several days, dehydration may occur.

6
7
9
10
16
44
91
95
99

Dislocation of bones: Dislocation may often be confirmed by the peculiar protrusion or angle of bones at various joints, especially joints with sockets such as where the arm joins the body. Relocating bones should not

13

be attempted by anyone unfamiliar with the process; the dislocated member should be taped or tied into an immobile position. G-Jo pressure-point stimulation does not replace standard Western first-aid or emergency techniques.

Dizziness (also see: Seasickness; Travel sickness; Vertigo; etc.): an unpleasant sensation of reeling, falling and disorientation. Sudden dizziness may indicate a more severe underlying condition.
10
37
38
65
77
79
81

Drowning (suffocation and asphyxia by fluids): This is an emergency/death-pending condition. G-Jo pressure-point stimulation does not replace standard Western first-aid or emergency techniques such as artificial ventilation (mouth-to-mouth resuscitation) etc. *Get medical help immediately.* Even if the victim appears to be normal afterwards, it is important for him to get medical attention since the possibility of infection, pneumonia and/or shock exists.
6
8
10
12
115

Drowsiness: see Bioenergy control centers; Sleep control centers; etc.

Drug abuses (also see: Intoxication; Poisoning by mouth; etc.): the improper use of prescribed medication or street drugs such as hallucinogens, etc. No G-Jo pressure-point stimulation should be done except in strictly emergency situations. *Get medical help immediately,* or contact a "hotline" agency such as exists in many urban centers. The telephone operator should have that information.
111

Dysentery (also see: Diarrhea; Gastrointestinal system; etc.): an easily spread disease
7
9

usually found in tropical, overcrowded conditions. It originates in contaminated food and/or water. There are several types of dysentery, and their symptoms include severe abdominal pain, frequent bowel movements (perhaps 25 or 30 per day – or more), loose to liquid stool, usually flecked with blood, pus and/or mucus. Children are most affected by this dangerous disease which is often confused with cholera. And, like cholera, *medical help is urgently required.*

10
16
44
91
95

Dyspepsia: see Indigestion; Flatulence; etc.

Dyspnea (also see: Asthma; Breath control centers; Hysteria; Mountain sickness; etc.): difficult or labored breathing sometimes symptomatic of an underlying disease or problem. It occurs when the capacity of the sufferer's breathing apparatus is temporarily unable to meet his body's demands, and often appears when breathing is reduced below 70% of maximum capacity. The sufferer may sense he is suffocating and panic, making the condition worse.

10
18

Ear (also see: Deafness, sudden, acute).

4	
13	
20	earache
45	
60	earache
64	
89	ear is damp and itchy
98	earache
100	ear is damp and itchy

Eczema: See Impetigo and eczema.

Edema (dropsy): an excessive accumulation of fluid in the body's tissues. Generally edema is a chronic problem.

7
9
48
57
72

Elbow (including "tennis elbow" — also see: Arm; etc.).

2
4
10
11
13
44
103

Electric shock (electrocution): This is an emergency condition. G-Jo pressure-point stimulation does not replace standard Western first-aid and emergency techniques. First, separate the victim from the source of electricity either by shutting off the power or by pushing the wire away with a wooden broom handle or other non-conductive material. Make sure your hands and feet are dry and that you are not standing on a conductive surface. *Get medical help immediately.*

8
15   fear and restlessness
18   victim is livid and
          corpse-like
21
115

Energy: see Bioenergy control centers; Stamina control centers; etc.

Epilepsy and epileptic seizures (also see: Convulsions; Convulsions in children; etc.): a brain disorder not clearly understood. There are a number of types of epileptic attacks; the most dramatic is the grand mal seizure. This may last from two to five minutes and generally includes loss of consciousness, loss of muscular control, rapid tensing and relaxing of the muscles of the extremities, etc. No G-Jo pressure-point stimulation should be used during a seizure; instead, try to help the sufferer avoid injuring himself, especially his tongue. If possible, place a cloth-wrapped stick between his teeth to prevent him from biting his tongue.

10
32
33
65
96
100

The sufferer should not immediately get up and move around, as this may trigger another seizure; instead he should be made as comfortable as possible with his clothing loosened.

Exhaustion, physical and/or mental (also see: Fatigue; Mental disturbances; Shock; etc.): the result of prolonged physical and/or mental stress or an excess of heat or cold or other unusual environmental factors. It is usually characterized by general listlessness, apprehension, weakness, dizziness, etc.

Exposure: see Exhaustion, physical and/or mental; Frostbite; Warm-up control centers; etc.

Eye (also see: Conjunctivitis): Beside diseases of the eye, there are three types of injuries that may occur:

   a. Injury to the eyelids and soft tissue surrounding the eye;

   b. Minor injury to the eye itself including chemical splashes, non-penetrating or non-embedded foreign objects, snow blindness, etc. Flush any chemical from the eye by holding the eyelid open while pouring a liberal amount of fresh water into the inner corner of the eye and letting the fluid flow over the eyeball. For removing foreign objects, the same procedure should be done or else gently pull the upper eyelid over the lower;

   c. Major injury to the eye. G-Jo pressure-point stimulation does not replace standard Western first-aid or emergency techniques. Major injuries primarily include embedded foreign objects or severe chemical or thermal burns. These problems threaten the victim's vision. *Get medical help immediately.* The eye should not be rubbed, nor should it be inspected until your hands are clean. A foreign body should *not* be removed with another foreign object such as a match or toothpick. And an embedded object should not be removed at all except by a doctor. Instead, wrap a bandage loosely around the head to protect the eye from further damage.

If the foreign object is not embedded, it may be lifted off gently with the corner of a clean handkerchief or tissue.

Face (including facial neuralgia, etc.—also see: Head; and specific areas, such as: Ear; Eye; Mouth: etc.).

1
2
4
5
13
38

Fainting (syncope—also see: Apoplexy; Dizziness; Exhaustion; Heart attack, heart failure; Unconsciousness; etc.): a state of unconsciousness or semiconsciousness resulting from a diminished supply of blood to the brain. Fear, shocking news, or any number of other factors can cause fainting. G-Jo pressure-point stimulation does not replace standard Western first-aid or emergency techniques.

12
15 due to fear and anxiety
34 with symptoms of
     hysteria
39
40 signs of heart attack
54
68
115

Getting blood back to the head is the immediate goal, either by seating the victim with his head between his knees or laying him flat with his head lower than the rest of his body. *Get medical help immediately.*

Fatigue (also see: Bioenergy control centers; Exhaustion, physical and/or mental; Stamina control centers; etc.): tiredness and lack of energy due to physical and/or mental exertion. Generally less serious than exhaustion, it is a substantial, though temporary, loss of strength.

9
21
54
97

Fear control centers: (also see: Anxiety; Fainting; Fear in children; Hysteria; etc.): a physical and/or mental reaction to a real or imagined situation. Individuals react differently and show different symptoms; sometimes the digestive tract reacts, other times there is a need to urinate or defecate, etc.

4
9
15
16
35
37
42
60
62   sudden, extreme fright
69   hysteria, panic
77
81
88
91
96
97
99

Fear in children (also see: Fear control centers; etc.).

35
69
88

Fever control centers: Fever is that state of bodily temperature beyond the normal 98.6° F. or 37° C. It is a defense mechanism; the body produces an inhospitable climate for "intruders," foreign bodies, parasites, etc., in an effort to remove their threat or to "neutralize" them. It is a natural process and may be symptomatic of many problems.

For high fever, scrape both sides of the spinal column gently with a spoon (after the back has been moistened with soapy water or vegetable oil) until the skin is a purplish color.

4
12
16   without sweating
61
101
104
also:
Hold ice on the pads of the big toes
Massage thumbs and pads of big toes
Massage the temples
Massage between the eyes and directly above the nose

Fingers: see Hand.

Fits: see Convulsions; Convulsions in children; Epilepsy and epileptic seizures; etc.

Flatulence (also see: Abdomen, lower; Indigestion; Gastrointestinal system; etc.): the presence of excessive gas in the stomach, intestines or anywhere in the gastrointestinal

7
9
72
74
85

system. Generally this is caused by dietary imbalances, anxiety or other minor digestive problems although it may be symptomatic of more serious or chronic problems.

93
108

Flu: see Colds and influenza.

Food poisoning: see Poisoning by mouth (oral poisoning); Poisoning, food; etc.

Foot (including ankle, toes, etc.—also see: Leg).

5
7
9
13
17
46
48
58
67
68
69
70
72 especially ankle
92 especially toes, if damp and itchy
104

Forearm (also see: Arm; Elbow; Hand; etc.).

2
10
12
13
18
33
37
39
72
76
77
116

Fracture (broken bone—also see specific area where the fracture has occurred such as Arm, etc.): a broken or splintered bone. G-Jo pressure-point stimulation does not replace standard Western first-aid or emergency techniques such as splints, casts, or other im-

26
42

mobilizing wrappings and coverings. But illustrated point no. 42, used throughout the time of healing, may help the fractured bone knit quickly and correctly.

Frostbite (including: Chilblain; Immersion Foot; Pernio; and Trench Foot—also see: Bioenergy control centers; Skin; Warm-up control centers; and specific areas affected, etc.): the result of prolonged exposure to damp or dry cold. The most severe condition is frostbite, where the tissue of the affected part of the body is destroyed by freezing. Blood circulation is stopped to the affected area; unless rapidly treated, this will become gangrenous and amputation may be required.

2
20   right side only, if skin is red and shiny
20   left side only, if skin is blue
27
28
29
30

The first signs are greyish or yellow-white spots on the skin; generally there will be numbness rather than pain. Long periods of inactivity and tight clothing increase the possibility of frostbite. The very young and the old, especially those with circulation problems, are the most susceptible. In a crisis situation (e.g., being lost in snow or frigid weather), walk around a fixed point such as a tree to keep the body warm and blood circulating. Aimless walking makes getting help difficult if there is another person who knows your approximate location.

Currently there is general agreement among authorities that immediate thawing in warm water as soon as the threat of refreezing is past is the best choice. But it will be painful. Never rub a frostbitten area, even with snow. *Get medical help immediately.*

Gall bladder (also see: Flatulence; Indigestion; etc.): a hollow organ located near the liver, in the upper right-hand quarter of the stomach-abdomen area, just beneath the rib-

1
7
9
13

cage. Its function is the accumulation and storage of mucus and bile. Pain or discomfort in that part of the upper abdomen, especially after eating, could indicate gall bladder or liver problems.

Gas, intestinal and/or stomach: see Flatulence.

Gastrointestinal system (also see: Abdomen, lower and upper; Flatulence; Indigestion; Stomach; etc.): the stomach and intestinal portions of the digestive tract.

7
9
13

Genital weakness, pain and/or dysfunction: see Gonorrhea; Sexual organs; etc.

genitourinary

Genitourinary system (also see: Bladder; Cystitis; Stricture of urine; Urinary control centers; etc.): the system whose job is the excretion of urine; it includes the kidneys, urinary bladder, ureters and urethra.

6
7
17
20
24
35
36
54
68
69

Gingivitis (bleeding gums, unhealthy gums —also see: Mouth; etc.): a condition which may be disease-linked, although more often it arises from improper and irregular care of the gums and teeth.

13
53
67
74

Goiter: an enlargement of the thyroid gland.

63

Gonorrhea (also see: Sexual organs; etc.): a venereal disease primarily involving the mucous membranes of the genitourinary tract and/or the rectum. Sometimes the eye is involved, as well. Its symptoms include painful urination, pus seepage from the urinary tract, and various genitourinary infections. Gonorrhea is primarily spread by sexual intercourse. *Get medical help immediately* both

19
20
68
72
83

for treatment and to help stop the spread of this disease.

Gout: a recurrent attack of acute arthritis that mostly strikes the big toe. The main symptom is mild to excruciating pain in or about the big toe. Sometimes crystal formations are found along the edges of the ear. Gout is caused by the improper metabolism of uric acid and may be triggered by an excess of wine or various rich foods.

35
48
58
74

Gunshot wounds: see Pain; Shock; Wounds; and specific areas of the body affected; etc. Gunshot wounds are often deceiving; they may look small, with little or no bleeding, but are nearly always more serious than they appear. *Get medical help immediately.* It is standard practice to report gunshot wounds to legal authorities. Not to do so might place you in serious legal difficulty.

Hand (including fingers—also see: Arm; Forearm; Wrist; etc.).

4	
10	
12	including fingers
13	
18	especially thumb
26	fingernail torn or crushed
38	
40	including wrist
61	
77	
79	
116	

Hangover (also see: Flatulence; Indigestion; Intoxication; etc.): the disagreeable aftereffects from drug or alcohol abuse. Its symptoms often include nausea, headache, indigestion, diarrhea, etc.

7
9
46

Hay Fever: see Allergies, non-specific; Eye; Nasal congestion (catarrh); Sneezing control centers; etc. Hay fever is a catchall term to describe a loosely knit group of allergic reactions triggered by pollination of various plants or weeds.

Head (also see: Ear; Eye; Face; Headache; Mouth; Neck; Whiplash; etc.): Any injury to the head is potentially dangerous. Signs of shock should be carefully watched for as well as signs of concussion. Fracture of the skull should be suspected, especially if there are differences between the size of the pupils, or bleeding from the nose, ears, and/or mouth. Keep the victim quiet and *get medical help immediately*.

1
2
4
9
10
12
13
15
21
69
88
97   if death seems near
103
105

Headaches (also see: Head; Migraine; Pain; etc.): may be symptomatic of many problems and diseases. If headache persists, or is a frequent problem, get medical help.

1
4
5
9
10
12
13
15   anxiety headache
17
38
59
64
67
68
69   top of head
75
80A   above eyes
81
87   mental strain
98
99
101   severe headache
106

44

Heart (also see: Angina pectoris; Chest; Heart attack, heart failure; etc.).

Heart attack, heart failure (also see: Angina pectoris; Cardiac arrest; Chest; Heart; Pain; Tachycardia; etc.): a major disturbance of the heart caused by either blockage of a coronary artery (heart attack) or inadequate pumping of the heart (heart failure). Symptoms of heart attack include severe pain or crushing pressure beneath the breastbone (sternum), a feeling of apprehension, shortness of breath, profuse sweating, and nausea and/or vomiting. The pain may first appear on the left side of the upper body before moving into the chest.

Symptoms of heart failure include edema (swelling of hands and feet), bluish-purple coloring of the skin, lips, fingernails, ears, etc., chest pains, anxiety and shortness of breath especially when lying down.

Get medical help immediately, and do not consume food or water when any heart disturbance is suspected.

Heartburn (including bile in the throat—also see: Chest; Heart attack, heart failure; Indigestion; Pain; etc.): A sudden dull-to-sharp, cutting pain in the chest area; it may be accompanied by burping, belching and/or raising acrid, bilious fluid.

Heat (body too hot): see Exhaustion, physical and/or mental; Overheating; Sunburn; Sunstroke; etc.

Heat rash (miliaria, "prickly heat"—also see: Hives and rash; Skin; etc.): an inflammation of the skin whose sores consist of raised, watery sacs usually in the folds of the skin. Often accompanied by a prickly, tingling sensation, it is mostly a summertime or tropical condition.

2	
9	
13	

Hemorrhage (bleeding—also see: Bleeding, arterial; **Bleeding, venous; Concussion; Menstruation;** Nosebleed; Wounds; and specific body areas affected; etc.): Blood flows through vessels such as veins and arteries, carrying oxygen and food to the cells and carrying away waste. If something happens to rupture the vessels, blood escapes; or disease may allow the blood to escape through unruptured vessels (diapedisis). Both are considered as hemorrhage; if enough blood escapes, death occurs. Arterial bleeding must be stopped immediately.

Bleeding from the mouth, rectum or nonmenstrual bleeding from the vagina may indicate internal hemorrhage. Other signs of bleeding may include weak or rapid pulse, cold and clammy skin, dull eyes, dilated pupils slow to respond to light, anxiety, excessive thirst, nausea and/or vomiting. Coma lasting more than six hours, stiffness of the neck coupled with cerebral dysfunction (such as unharmonious eye movements) with or without other symptoms of internal bleeding may indicate cerebral hemorrhage.

Any internal hemorrhaging is a dangerous condition. *Get medical help immediately.*

4	severe, bright red blood
9	
11	
13	
19	
20	left side only, if dark, venous blood is flowing, plus
21	ten minutes later if there is slow bleeding from the nose and ears
28	cerebral hemorrhage
43	
44	bright, red blood
49	
79	
99	cerebral hemorrhage
103	
110	arterial or venous bleeding
111	bleeding anywhere in the body

Hemorrhoids (piles—also see: Pain; Rectum; etc.): an enlarged, expanded vein in the lower rectal and/or anal wall. Complications may include inflammation, bleeding, pain and/or itching and possibly clotting (thrombosis).

5	pain
8	
65	
72	bleeding hemorrhoids
83	
99	

Permanently curing hemorrhoids usually means a change in diet, toilet habits and/or mental attitudes.

Hepatitis: see Liver. This is an inflammation of the liver which is dangerous and may be communicable. *Get medical help immediately.*

Hernia (rupture—also see: Abdomen, lower; etc.): an abnormal protrusion of the intestine through the abdominal muscle wall or cavity. Hernia is often caused by lifting an excessive weight or improperly hoisting a load. Ordinarily, a small-to-large bulge will appear somewhere upon the abdomen; and there may be some pain. The ultimate danger lies in the possibility of the source of blood to the protruding bowel being cut off.

7
9
50
62
68

Herpes simplex virus (also see: Shingles).

114

Hiccough (hiccup) **control center**: With older persons, especially, hiccoughs are often associated with hardening of the arteries (arteriosclerosis).

1
6
10
31
45   massage downward
95
96
97

High blood pressure: see Hypertension.

Hip (also see: Buttocks; etc.).

5
7
9
41
50
62
63
67

Hives and rash (urticaria—also see: Allergies, non-specific; Skin; etc.): sudden or rapid appearance of intensive, itching welts on the skin. They may appear in crops over wide areas of the body, tend to last a day or so,

2
23
106

and are generally associated with allergic reactions.

In severe cases, hives may affect the mucous membrane areas; edema may constrict the vocal area (glottis), creating possibly fatal distress.

Hunger control centers: not to be used as a regular dietary aid, but only to help temporarily tide you over until food is available.

Hypertension (high blood pressure): Its symptoms are as vague as the origin of the disease. Besides increased blood pressure, there may be dizziness, fatigue, insomnia, palpitations, weakness and headaches, etc. Massaging the rear edges at the back of the ears is often helpful.

Hyperventilation (also see: Anxiety; etc.): deep, rapid overbreathing, often associated with fear or anxiety. Overbreathing produces a temporary imbalance in the blood (too alkaline, not enough carbon dioxide). Its symptoms include dizziness, tingling, crawling and/or burning sensations on the skin and possibly fainting (syncope).

Breathing into a paper bag held tightly over the mouth and nose may help restore a proper gaseous and chemical balance in the blood.

Hypoglycemia (low blood sugar—also see: Diabetes mellitus; Spleen and pancreas; etc.): a condition about which little is known, but it is thought by some nutrition authorities to affect millions. The problem is too much insulin and/or not enough "blood sugar," which may trigger insulin shock in severe cases. Its symptoms may be similar to diabetes mellitus, a problem with which it is often confused.

Hypotension (low blood pressure): a condition mostly associated with other underlying problems or diseases. 16 110

Hysteria (also see: Anxiety; Fear control centers; etc.): panicky, severe fear whose symptoms may include sweating, palpitations, tension and fatigue, irrationality, undefined terror and sense of impending calamity, etc. Urinary or bowel urgency may occur. While hysteria is common with prepubescent and pubescent children, it may indicate problems of a severe nature in adults. *Get medical help immediately.* 15 34 69 99 also deeply massage hands for several minutes

Impetigo and eczema (also see: Skin, etc.): skin disorders whose symptoms are crusty, yellowish formations and pustules (impetigo) or drier, more reddened lesions (eczema); or they may look similar. 2 3 5 7 35 40 61

Indigestion (also see: Flatulence, Gastrointestinal system; Stomach; etc.): a temporary disorder of the digestive tract often caused by overeating, alcohol abuse or nervousness, etc. Its symptoms include flatulence and discomfort in the upper or lower abdomen, etc. 6 7 9 31 46 95 96 108

Infection: the "invasion" of the body by various organisms such as hostile bacteria or viruses. 113

Influenza: see Colds and influenza.

Injuries: see Wounds; also see specific area of

injury such as: Arm; Hand; Leg; and associated symptoms.

Insanity: see Mental disturbances.

Insect bites and stings: see Bites, animal, human and insect; Stings, bee and wasp; Stings, scorpion; etc.

Insensibility: see Fainting (syncope); Unconsciousness; etc.

Insomnia: sleeplessness and mild restlessness; prolonged difficulty in getting to sleep. Often you may have slept lightly, or even deeply, without realizing it.

6
10
15
18
35
40
46
59
64
84
97

Insulin reactions: see Diabetes (diabetes mellitus); Hypoglycemia.

Intestinal problems: see Constipation (costiveness); Diarrhea; Dysentery; Gastrointestinal system; Flatulence; Indigestion; Pain; etc.

Intoxication (also see: Hangover; Indigestion; etc.): mild or severe poisioning from the abuse of alcohol, medication, or drugs. Its symptoms range from mild euphoria to violent mental and/or physical reactions, and, rarely, death. In the event that an intoxicated person is the victim of an accident, great care should be taken since he may not realize the full extent of his injuries. *Get medical help immediately,* and keep him warm in cold, wet weather.

49
90   after the intoxication

Jaundice (also see: Liver; etc.): yellowing of the skin or mucous membranes, and secretions with bile pigment. Jaundice may occur from a number of causes, but is generally disease-linked. The liver is primarily or secondarily affected; this is the bile-producing organ.

10
17
23
86
93
98
109

Jaw, lower (also see: Mouth; Toothache; etc.)

1
4
5
13
24
56

Kidneys (also see: Back, lower and/or upper).

20
69

Knee (also see: Foot; Leg; Thigh; etc.).

3
9
57
62
63

Laryngitis (also see: Bronchitis; Colds and influenza; Respiratory problems; Throat; etc.): an inflammation of the larynx or voice box which causes a hoarseness or inability to vocalize sound. Chronic or acute, it may be caused by a number of factors.

1
11
12
13
56

Leg (also see: Foot; Knee; Thigh: etc.).

3
5
7
9
62

Lethargy: see Bioenergy control centers; Sleep control centers; Stamina control centers; etc.

Lightheadedness (also see: Dizziness; Fainting; Vertigo; etc.).

60

Lips (also see: Face; Head; Mouth; etc.).

13

Liver (also see: Gall bladder; Indigestion; Jaundice; Spleen and pancreas; etc.): the largest gland or secreting organ in the body. Its functions are not totally understood, but it plays a major role in the digestive process. Symptoms of a liver disorder may include pain and/or discomfort behind the bottom of the rib cage and are sometimes confused with problems of the gall bladder. 17 35 66 93 94

Lockjaw: see Tetanus.

Low blood pressure: see Hypotension.

Low blood sugar: see Hypoglycemia.

Lumbago (also see: Back, lower and/or upper; Pain; Sciatica; etc.): aching in the lower to middle back region. 1 3 5 7 9 11 13 19 24 38 49 65 111

Lungs (also see: Bronchitis; Chest; Respiratory system; etc.). 1 97 107

Malaria (also see: Fever control centers; Sweating control centers; etc.): a generally chronic, recurring disease accompanied by fever, involuntary spasms, chills and sweating, etc. 20 33 38 88 93 96

Man-o-war burns (also see: Burns and scalds, chemical; Pain; etc.): a tropical and subtropical seashore pest that may cause severe burn injuries—and occasionally death—to unwary bathers. Its long tentacles (up to 50 feet) contain a powerful acid that clings to the skin. Its effect has been likened to an electric shock that doesn't stop. Two steps should be taken:

    a. Remove the acid; use either alcohol or, better, a mild solution of ammonia;

    b. Neutralize the burn; use ammonia, baking soda, meat tenderizer, or over-the-counter antacid liquids or gels, and pat onto the affected area.

Measles: an acute infectious disease characterized first by inflammation of the mucous membranes of the eyes and air passages, then by eruption of a rash after three or four days. Typically the rash first appears behind the ears, on the face, the chest, and/or the abdomen. Cough, plus conjunctivitis and/or tiny, grey-white spots on red bases on the inner jaw should lead you to suspect measles. During the course of the disease, protect the eyes from bright light. 44   after rash has erupted

Memory control centers (also see: Apoplexy; etc.): Any sudden onset of difficulty with remembering could mean a severe underlying problem such as apoplexy (stroke) or cerebral hemorrhage. *Get medical help immediately.* 1
10
78

Meningitis: an inflammation of the brain and/or spinal cord caused by any number of factors. There are several types of meningitis, at least one of which is contagious. Symptoms of meningitis may include headache, aching with pain radiating down the neck, stiff neck, vomiting and nausea, sore throat, upper respiratory infection, pain in and about one eye, drooping eyelid(s). A very serious disease, *it is urgent to get medical help immediately.* 12

Menstruation (also see: Abdomen, lower; Pain; Sexual organs; etc.).

6
7
8
10
14
16
27
35
68   excessive flow of menses
87   premenstrual pain and tension

Mental disturbances (also see: Anxiety; Fear control centers; Hysteria; etc.): Actions and indications of mental disturbance can range from mild depression to anger, irrationality, and suicidal attempts. According to oriental theory, mental disturbances are generally organ-linked and are yet another indication of the body's bioenergy being out of balance and harmony.

9   depression
16
31   irrationality
32   suicidal tendencies
47   depression
62   irrationality
76   depression
79
95
96
98   suicidal tendencies
99

Migraine (also see: Headache; etc.): a particularly severe headache, often associated with a malfunctioning liver by nutritional authorities. It is characterized by periodic, rapid onsets that often center in or around one or both eyes and may be accompanied by other painful, unpleasant symptoms. Vomiting, nausea, loss of appetite and strength are not uncommon.

1
13
15
17
18
66
101
106
115
also massage the inner half (side closest to the second toe) of the big toe and/or the lower earlobes; or plunge hands into very hot or very cold water

Miliaria: see Heat rash.

Mosquito bites: see Bites, animal, human and insect.

Motion sickness: see Dizziness; Seasickness; Travel sickness; Vertigo; etc.

Mountain sickness (hypoxia, altitude sickness): difficult, labored breathing (dyspnea), headache, lightheadedness, and other reactions resulting from a lack of oxygen to the tissues, coupled with lower atmospheric pressure. In severe cases death results; in less severe cases, the aftereffects may last up to 48 hours and include headache, nausea, vomiting, and lethargy. It is urgent to get back to a more normal atmospheric pressure and to bring more oxygen to the tissues. *Get medical help immediately.* 47 82

Mouth (also see: Dental work; Face; Gingivitis; Head; Jaw, lower; Lips; Tongue; Toothache; etc.). 13 20 49 65 102 sores in mouth

Mumps: an acute, painful and contagious viral disease. Its symptoms are generally an enlargement of one or both salivary glands—especially the parotid gland (located in front of and below the ear)—but may include attack on other tissues such as the testicles, pancreas, etc. 4 13 33 89

Muscles (also see: Cramps, muscular; Sprains, muscular; Strains, muscular; etc.). 62

Nasal congestion (catarrh—also see: Colds and influenza; Sinusitis; etc.): an inflammation of the nasal passages' mucous membranes combined with a mucus discharge. 1 12 13 60 75 79 98 99 106 112

Nausea (also see: Dizziness; Indigestion; Sea-sickness; Travel sickness; Vertigo; etc.): a feeling of discomfort, impending vomiting, and an aversion to food and/or liquids.

3
7
9
18

Neck (also see: Whiplash; etc.).

1
2
13
21
23
25
29
35
43
47
50
80B
98
100
103
104
106
116

Nervousness (also see: Anxiety; Fear control centers; Mental disturbances; etc.): a state of mental and/or physical disarray, characterized by a lack of mental poise and composure, restlessness, impulsive and/or irrational behavior, purposeless activity, etc.

4
10
13
15
17
32   nervousness in children
35
45   massage downward
99

Neuralgia (also see: Pain; specific areas affected, such as Arm; Hand; etc.): aching sensitivity or brief, stabbing pains along the course of a nerve.

5   pain
13
24

Night sweating (also see: Sweating control centers; etc.): drenching perspiration during sleep. This condition may be associated with feverish diseases or mental disturbances, etc.

70

Nightmares (especially affecting children—also see: Anxiety; Hysteria; Nervousness; etc.): frightening dreams.

88

Nosebleed (epistaxis): a nasal hemorrhage which may be minor and simple or linked to more serious problems such as concussion.

1
3
13
23
32
60
74
79
81
82
98
100
106

Numbness (also see: Unconsciousness; etc.): local or general insensitivity (anesthesia), often coupled with sluggishness, etc.

45

Ovaries: see Menstruation; Sexual organs; etc.

Overheating (if you are too warm from exertion, etc.—also see: Night sweating; Sweating control center): Relax for a few minutes, then:
   a. Massage the pad of each big toe;
   b. Plunge wrists into cool water;
   c. Take a warm shower or bath; pat partly dry and finish your drying by evaporation.

Pain control centers (also see: Headache; Neuralgia; specific portions of body affected, such as Arm; Hand; etc.): Pain is one of the body's first lines of communication and defense and may arise from conditions in parts of the body away from the pain site. For chronic recurring pain, get medical help.

1	general
2	pain in joints
3	lower back
4	chest, ribs
5	general
7	lower body, testicles, lower back, menstrual
9	middle, lower body
10	arm, armpit, shoulder
13	upper body, head, feet
24	face
27	menstrual
29	upper back
38	middle back
40	between the ribs

Pain control centers *continued*

47	neck, shoulder, upper back
48	testicles, lower back
49	general, face, intercostal pain
58	testicles, lower back
59	lower back and abdomen together
60	"writer's cramp"
61	chest, ribs, arm, shoulder and loins
63	general
68	penis, uterus
73	inner thigh, genitals
75	
77	general
79	hand
87	general
88	ear
101	eye
115	general
116	loin to navel

Panic: see Anxiety; Fear control centers; Hysteria; etc.

Paralysis (also see: Numbness; etc.): loss of sensation and muscle function due to injury to the nervous system and/or disease-linked destruction of the nervous connections. Partial or complete paralysis may even be triggered by psychological problems and conditions such as hysteria. Paralysis may affect specific areas or half the body (hemiplegia) or more. *Get medical help immediately.*

4	infantile paralysis
23	
41	
50	
63	
72	lower limbs
75	
89	facial paralysis
95	
98	hemiplegia
99	hemiplegia

Paralysis, infantile: see Paralysis.

Peritonitis (also see: Abdomen, lower; etc.): an inflammation of the wall of the abdominal cavity resulting from any number of sources such as a ruptured appendix or wound, etc. Its symptoms include severe abdominal pain (often intensified by movement) and abdominal distention. The more severe the problem, the more distended the abdomen may be. Vomiting and/or diarrhea may be present in

94	
96	

the early stages; fever, chills, and rapid pulse usually follow. The sufferer appears very sick—which he is.

Peritonitis is a complication of an underlying problem or condition; foods and fluids should not be given. This is an extremely serious problem and, untreated, will usually lead to death. *Get medical help immediately.*

Pleurisy (also see: Chest; Pain; Pneumonia; etc.): an inflammation of the inner chest cavity sometimes accompanying infections of the lungs and/or chest areas. The primary symptom is pain, either mild or severe, while breathing. Pleurisy is generally symptomatic of a more serious underlying condition. *Get medical help immediately.*

Pneumonia (also see: Chest; Pleurisy; etc.): an inflammation of the air sacs in the lungs. There are a number of forms of pneumonia, and each represents a potentially dangerous threat. Often pneumonia is a complication of other problems or diseases. Colds and influenza, chronic alcoholism, malnutrition, exposure, and foreign matter in the respiratory tract are only a few of the conditions that may lead to this disorder.

Although pneumonia may be either bacterial or non-bacterial, symptoms are the same and include shaking chills, sharp pain in either or both sides of the chest, cough with a pinkish-to-rusty sputum, fever and headache, etc. *Get medical help immediately.*

Poison ivy, oak or sumac (also see: Skin; etc.): a plant poisoning that primarily affects the skin, but may also affect various mucous membranes such as eyes, nose, etc. The most typical symptoms include red, swollen skin and furiously itching, small blisters. The affected area should first be washed with hot water, soap and alcohol. Learning to recognize the offending plants will be of great future help since each exposure may render you increasingly sensitive to the irritating agent in the plants.

Poisoning by mouth (oral poisoning—also see: Abdomen, lower and/or upper; Gastrointestinal system; Poisoning, food; Stomach: etc.): Speed is of the utmost importance when dealing with oral poisoning; it is often an emergency/death-pending condition.

There are numerous symptoms of oral poisoning, depending upon the poison and the amount (see notes in the margin). G-Jo pressure-point stimulation does not replace standard Western first-aid or emergency techniques. *Get medical help immediately, and contact the poison control center in a major hospital.*

13	vomiting and purging; face is pale, blue and with cold sweating
18	restlessness, exhaustion, nausea; face swollen, pale and cold, covered with sweat; repeat stimulation each half hour
24	burning in the throat
50	violent abdominal pains
51	throat feels fiery; hard to swallow; face is swollen, pale, wretched
52	
53	
77	

Poisoning, carbon monoxide: Carbon monoxide is the lethal by-product of fuel combustion. Automobile engines or acetylene torches used in tightly enclosed areas are the usual offenders. The victim must be moved immediately into fresh air with minimal exertion on his part.

17
18
78

Symptoms of carbon monoxide poisoning include dizziness, intense headache, full pulse, possible vomiting, pulsing temples, possible muscular twitching, dilated, widely-opened pupils, drowsiness, rapid breathing, and lips that are blue, pale or pink, with bluish-red patches on the skin. G-Jo pressure-point stimulation does not replace standard

Western first-aid or emergency techniques. *Get medical help immediately, and contact the poison control center in a major hospital.*

Poisoning, food (also see: Abdomen, lower and/or upper; Gastrointestinal system; Poisoning by mouth; Stomach; etc.): a broadly-based category of symptoms covering both bacterial and non-bacterial poisoning from poorly preserved or prepared foods as well as food already contaminated before leaving its native environment (notably seafood).

18   restlessness, exhaustion, burning pains, nausea; face is swollen, pale, cold and sweaty

53

104 mild to moderate

105 if more severe

    Its symptoms may include any possible digestive tract reaction as well as possible damage to the central nervous system. In severe cases, every system of the body may be affected or death may occur. Symptoms of untreated food poisoning may last as long as several months. This is a serious problem; G-Jo pressure-point stimulation does not replace standard Western first-aid or emergency techniques. *Get medical help immediately, and contact the poison control center in a major hospital.*

Poisoning, ptomaine: see Poisoning by mouth (oral poisoning); Poisoning, food; etc.: an outdated term that generally refers to food poisoning.

"Possession by devils" (also see: Mental disturbances; etc.): In cultures or subcultures that believe in devilish possession, symptoms such as marked change in behavior—invariably unpleasant—antisocial actions, rapid changes in physical appearance, etc., are thought to be signs of such possession. In short, any sort of rapid change that makes the sufferer more or less unrecognizable in action and/or appear-

78

ance to friends of long standing is suspect. Classical schizophrenia, brain tumors, and numerous other mental and/or physical disorders may exhibit similar symptoms.

Prostate (also see: Sexual organs; etc.): the organ surrounding the neck of the urinary bladder in the male. Symptoms of prostate problems often include itching and burning in and around the front of the urethral canal (urethral meatus) of the penis, especially in the morning, and pain in the groin and/or lower back region.

6
7
8
9
19
20
24
72

Puncture wounds: see Tetanus; Wounds; specific areas of the body affected; etc.

Queasiness: see Dizziness; Nausea; Vertigo; etc.

Rabies: see Bites, animal, human, and insect. Untreated rabies is usually fatal; *get medical help immediately.*

Rash: see Hives and rash (urticaria); Measles; Skin; etc.

Rectum (also see: Gastrointestinal system; Gonorrhea; Hemorrhoids; etc.): the lowest part of the large intestine ending at the anus.

5
24
65

Respiratory system (also see: Bronchitis; Chest; Lungs; Pneumonia; etc.): the system of the body pertaining to the breathing apparatus.

1
10
11
13
97
107
112

Restlessness (also see: Anxiety; Fear control center; Mental disturbances; Poisoning (of all types); Shock; etc.): aimless activity more

15
16
97

62

severe than the sort usually associated with boredom. Often restlessness is indicative of an underlying physical and/or mental problem. *Get medical help immediately.*

Retching: see Vomiting and retching.

Rheumatism: no G-Jo pressure-point stimulation to be used.

Rhinitis: see Nasal congestion; Sinusitis.

Scalds: see Burns and scalds.

Sciatica (also see: Back, lower; Buttocks; Hip; Leg; Lumbago; Pain; etc.): pain and tenderness along the sciatic nerve, ranging from the lower back down (distally) as far as the foot.

3 63
4 75
5 80B
7 83
9
19
24
38
41
42
57
62

Scorpion stings: see Stings, scorpion.

Seasickness (also see: Dizziness; Nausea; Travel sickness; Vertigo; Vomiting and retching; etc.): a minor to severe feeling of illness, nausea and queasiness, often accompanied by vomiting and retching, dizziness, loss of appetite, etc. It is primarily associated with the motion of a boat or ship at sea, but may be triggered by the rocking of an unstable platform. While this unpleasant condition might last as long as several days in an unstable site, it is usually only a temporary problem that eases as your equilibrium becomes more atuned to the surrounding environment or as soon as you reach a firm, stable location. Drink no alcohol.

3
7
9
10
31

Sedation and tranquilization control centers (also see: Anxiety; Nervousness; etc.): for minor nervousness not associated with severe problems or mental disturbances of a serious nature.

13
17

Sexual organs (also see: Gonorrhea; Prostate; etc.): including the penis, testicles, and related parts of the male reproductive system; and the vagina, ovaries, and womb (uterus) of the female system.

2   uterus and ovaries
6
7   esp. impotence, frigidity
8
9
19
41   impotence, frigidity
52
54
57   impotence
68   pain in penis
70
73
81
111

Shingles (herpes zoster): a particularly painful infection of the central nervous system. Its symptoms include small eruptions and neuralgic pain, especially around the waist. Shingles most often occurs in persons over fifty years old.

114

Shock (also see: Unconsciousness; etc.): a gradual to rapid collapse of the circulatory system's functions wherein a continuing deficiency of blood reaches the peripheral tissues; *this should not be confused with electric shock (electrocution).*

A victim in shock may be conscious, semiconscious or unconscious; he may be responsive or not, but his perception is usually impaired and he seems numb and apathetic. Pain may or may not be present. Thirst, especially when accompanied by other symptoms, may be an indication of this

10
15
18
21   severe shock
69   percussion with knuckle:
      repeat 12 times
103
115
116

dangerous condition. Restlessness is common, as are pallor and/or sweating. The pulse is generally faint and rapid; hyperventilation often occurs. Shock may be fatal; *get medical help immediately.*

Shock is symptomatic of an underlying condition such as injured tissue or, less frequently, illness. It may occur immediately after trauma or injury or several hours later; it may be triggered by rough handling, excessive cold, pain, loss of blood (hemorrhage), or for no special reason at all. Warmth is important to the victim, as is getting a proper flow of blood to his head. G-Jo pressure-point stimulation does not replace standard Western first-aid or emergency techniques.

Shock, electric: see Electric shock (electrocution).

Shock, emotional: see Fainting; Hysteria; etc.

Shoulder (also see: Neck; etc.).

1
2
4
10
11
13
21
29
35
43
47
61
62
72   joint
103
104
106
116

Sinusitis (problems of the sinuses—also see: Headache; Nasal congestion; etc.): inflammation of the sinus cavities in and around the nose and eyes. When a G-Jo pressure point is stimulated, there may be drainage.

1
12
13
46
80A
80B
112

Skin (also see: Acne; Impetigo and eczema; Hives and rash; Wounds; etc.).

2
3
4
27
28
40

Sleep control centers (also see: Anxiety; Bioenergy control centers; Insomnia; Mental disturbances; etc.): The temporary desire for excessive sleep is often a symptom of an underlying psychological problem and/or improper diet; rarely, it may be one of the several "sleeping sicknesses."

64
68
97

Sluggishness: see Bioenergy control centers; etc.

Small intestines: the organ which completes the digestion process, located between the stomach and the large intestines.

7
9
19

Smoke inhalation: see Asphyxia (suffocation).

Smoking control centers: To help temporarily ease your desire for tobacco, the first thing to do so is to take ten long, deep breaths (inhale through the nose, exhale through pursed lips), as slowly as possible. Many of your signals to light a cigarette are the body's subtle demand for air; the only time many smokers breathe properly and deeply is when smoking.

7
9
10
11
31
97

Besides stimulating the G-Jo pressure points, tugging and pinching each ear lobe may also be helpful; if you are trying to stop smoking, avoid the excessive use of alcohol or sweets as they may trigger the desire to smoke.

Snakebite (also see specific effects of snakebite, such as Hemorrhage; Hysteria; Shock; etc.): Actual cases of poisonous snakebite are quite rare; and of those, less than 20% of untreated cases are fatal.

First, make sure you have been bitten by a poisonous snake—or even bitten at all. Look for one or two fang punctures, as the pit viper (rattlesnake, moccasin and copperhead) is by far the more common bite. There may be bleeding; there will be pain and a harsh, stinging sensation. Make sure this is from a bite and not from an injury during a fall, etc.

The pit viper's (Family Crotalidae) poison causes damage (and death) from hemorrhage. Snakes of the Family Elapidae (coral snakes, cobras and kraits, etc.) have a poison that causes paralysis. Either of these conditions must be considered in an actual case of snakebite.

Slowing or stopping the dispersion of the poison is extremely important:

a. Tie a tourniquet or constricting band between the site of the bite and the heart; it should be firm-to-tight, but it must be loosened for a few moments every five minutes. The closer to the bite site the tourniquet is tied, the better.

b. Pack the punctured area, if possible, with freshwater ice slush (half water, half ice): the immersion should extend well above the bite site. This will help the poison disperse slowly and assist the body tissues to possibly absorb and assimilate the posion without serious trauma or damage.

c. If no ice is available, crush some earthworms and pat the extracted juice upon the puncture after it has been slightly opened with a sterilized knife or razor.

Do not drink alcohol. G-Jo pressure-point

19   immediately, for one minute; deep, hard pressure

20   left foot only; deep, hard pressure for one minute

67

stimulation does not replace standard Western first-aid or emergency techniques; *get medical help immediately.*

Sneezing control centers: Caused by irritation of the nasal nerves or overstimulation of the optic nerves by bright light, sneezing may be symptomatic of allergies or colds and influenza, etc.

11
80B
81
115

Sore throat: see Colds and influenza; Throat; etc.

Spasm, muscular: see Cramps and spasms, muscular; Muscles; Pain.

Spider bites: see Bites, spider.

Spleen and pancreas (also see Diabetes mellitus; Gall bladder; Liver; Stomach; etc.): Located in the upper left-hand quarter of the abdomen, beneath the left side of the rib cage, the spleen is the largest lymph gland of the body. Immediately beside the spleen is the pancreas, the gland responsible for the production of insulin, etc.

7
9
48
57
58
68
93
109

Sprains, muscular (also see: Muscles; Pain; Strains, muscular; specific areas of injury, such as Foot, Wrist, etc.): injuries to the soft tissues surrounding the joints. Sprains generally occur when the joint is forced into more extreme action than it is capable of handling. Keep stress away from the sprained area since the injury is sometimes a tearing or partial ripping of the ligaments, muscles and/or blood vessels of the affected area.

5   pain
41
54
62

Stage fright: see Anxiety; Nervousness; etc.

68

Stamina control centers (also see: Bioenergy control centers; Breath control centers): Stamina is aggressive energy, determination, endurance and "will power."

Stimulation: see Bioenergy control centers; Stamina control centers; etc.

Stings, bee and wasp (also see: Bites, animal, human and insect; Bites, spider; Shock; etc.): For stings from all flying insects, first remove the stinger by dragging a fingernail or edged utensil backwards against the stinger; do not pluck it out with a tweezers or squeeze the small bulb at its end because this will inject more venom into the puncture.

Bee stings may be treacherous, especially in the event of a massive attack by a colony or, rarely, by swarming bees; some individuals react violently, even fatally, to even one bee sting. The venom of bees is similar to that of the pit viper (Family Crotalidae). If you have a history of allergic reaction to bee or wasp stings, or show symptoms of illness, *get medical help immediately.*

Stings, scorpions (also see: Bites, animal, human and insect; Bites, spider; Stings, bee and wasp; etc.): Generally the sting of a scorpion is not serious and is seldom fatal. Most dangerously affected are infants and young children stung by one of the several varieties in southwestern North America. *Get medical help immediately* if symptoms of illness arise.

Stomach (also see: Abdomen, upper; Gall bladder; Gastrointestinal system; Indigestion; etc.): this dilated organ of the gastrointestinal system is located directly below the diaphragm.

Strains, muscular (including "charley horse" —also see: Muscles; Pain; Sprains, muscular; etc.): Muscular strains are much like sprains, except they usually occur away from the joint. With muscular strains, muscle fibers are stretched too far, sometimes even torn.

5   pain
62

Strength, loss of, or to temporarily regain: see Bioenergy control centers; Stamina control centers; etc.

Stricture of urine (also see: Cystitis; Gonorrhea; Urinary system; Urinary control centers): a condition where the kidneys continue to secrete urine, but the bladder passes only small amounts at a time, often accompanied by a sharp burning or cutting pain. This may be due to blockage and/or disease.

17
35
36
59
68
69
99

Stroke: see Apoplexy.

Stuttering control center.

84

Styes: see Boils, styes, and carbuncles.

Suffocation: see Asphyxia (suffocation).

Suicidal tendencies: see Mental disturbances.

Sunburn: see Burns and scalds (sunburn);

Sunstroke (also see: Burns and scalds; Exhaustion; etc.): Symptoms of sunstroke may include unconsciousness or semiconsciousness, hot, dry skin, high temperature, headache, dizziness, red face and skin. Before using G-Jo pressure-point stimulation, move the victim into the shade with his head and shoulders slightly elevated and his clothing loosened. Give cool or tepid water slowly, and *get medical help immediately.*

10
12
13
55   severe sunstroke
82

Sweating control centers (also see: Night sweating; Overheating; etc.): Before using G-Jo pressure-point stimulation, relax for a few minutes especially if sweating has been produced by hard, physical labor or exercise.
3
13
72

Syncope: see Fainting.

Tachycardia, paroxysmal (also see: Anxiety; Fear; Heart; Hysteria; etc.): a condition when the heartbeat rate suddenly and dramatically increases. An attack may last from minutes to days stopping as suddenly as it began. It may be associated with heart disease, but not necessarily. There may or may not be pain. *Get medical help immediately.*
9
15
37
42
60
81

Temper control centers: especially for sudden, irrational anger.
4
15
17
31
35
37
43
66
91

Tennis elbow: see Elbow.

Testicles, including crushed testicles (also see: Pain; Sexual organs; etc.): Injury to the testicles is one of the most painful and agonizing conditions that can happen to the male body; even a mild injury to the testicles may be completely debilitating.
5
7
9
48
58   severe injury
72

Tetanus (lockjaw—also see: Bites, animal, human and insect; Wounds): an infectious disease caused by a wound not exposed to oxygen. Any wound may result in tetanus infection; punctures and bites are notorious, especially where there is the presence of rust and/or fecal matter.
22
61
68   immediately after the skin is punctured and regularly afterwards

As tetanus progresses, spasms of the voluntary muscles occur and convulsions become frequent. Muscle stiffness after a puncture wound (any time between two and 50 days, but usually between five and ten days) should lead you to suspect tetanus, especially if you have had no inoculation against the disease within several years.

With tetanus, the jaw muscles will eventually lock, accompanied by a grotesque grimace or smile with raised eyebrows. Untreated tetanus is generally fatal. For any wound, if you have not had a recent tetanus vaccination, *get medical help immediately.*

Thigh (also see: Hip; Knee; Leg; Pain): the part of the leg from the pelvis to the knee.

3
41
62
73

Thirst control centers: A regular intake of fluids is vital to the body; it can exist for a much longer time without food than without water. In cases where an adequate supply of liquid does not replace lost fluid, dehydration may occur. In severe cases, shock may occur, as well. For any situation when dehydration is suspected, *get medical help immediately;* drinking water, alone, may not relieve the complications since an electrolytic change in the body may have occurred.

18
44
78
102
110

In the event of emergency conditions, several steps may be taken to temporarily relieve thirst aside from stimulating the G-Jo pressure point(s):

a. Place a small pebble in your mouth to generate saliva;

b. Gargle a small amount of the available remaining water, then spit it back into a container for future use;

c. Drink your own urine; it will not harm you as long as it is your own.

When water again becomes available, drink it slowly and only a few sips at a time.

Throat (also see: Colds and influenza; Tonsilitis; etc.).

1	
4	
11	
12	main point
13	
18	
20	
65	
99	

Toes: see Athlete's foot; Foot.

Tongue (also see: Mouth).

13	
49	swollen tongue
87	

Tonsilitis (also see: Throat; etc.): inflammation of the tonsils (small glands in the
throat). Its symptoms include chills, sore-
ness, rapidly rising temperature, difficulty in
swallowing, stiff neck, etc.

3
4
12
13
38
46
79
84

Toothache (also see: Dental work; Jaw, lower;
Mouth; Pain).

5		98
13		106
24		113
37		115
46	upper jaw	116
53		
56		
67		
72		
74	upper jaw	
82	esp. molars	

Tooth extraction, drilling, etc.: see Dental
work.

Torticollis (stiff neck, "wry neck"): see Neck;
Whiplash (neck injury).

Travel sickness (also see: Dizziness; Nausea;
Seasickness; Stomach; Vertigo; etc.): For any
sort of travel sickness (due to trains, cars,
airplanes, etc.), avoid alcohol.

3
7
9
10
31

Tumors: no G-Jo pressure-point stimulation
to be used.

Ulcers, intestinal (also see: Abdomen, lower and/or upper; Gastrointestinal system; etc.): lesions in the intestinal tract. Typical symptoms include nausea, vomiting and retching, diarrhea and black stools. *Get medical help immediately.*

4
7
9

Ulcers, peptic (especially duodenal and gastric—also see: Gastrointestinal tract; Stomach; etc.): lesions that form in the digestive tract and are often associated with stress. The symptoms include:

7
9
41   stomach, duodenal
85
86

   a. duodenal ulcers: "hunger" pains that are often associated with excess stomach acidity;
   b. gastric ulcers: "Sluggish stomach" from an underproduction of stomach acids.
Get medical help immediately if either sort of ulcer is suspected.

Unconsciousness, causes unknown (also see: Apoplexy; Asphyxia; Fainting; Heart attack, heart failure; etc.): the victim lacks an awareness of self and surroundings and gives little or no response to sensory input. Unconsciousness is always a serious problem; G-Jo pressure-point stimulation does not replace standard Western first-aid or emergency techniques. *Get medical help immediately.*

12   unconscious; face bright red
18   from head injury; no convulsions present

19
20   left foot only
21   any head injury; plus 18 with severe head injury, if death seems close? use each half hour until improvement, if medical help is not available; also general unconsciousness
26   unconsciousness from spinal concussion or injury
32
33   unconscious; violent convulsions
34   unconscious; face is pale; hysterical symptoms
68   general unconsciousness
115
116

Urinary control centers (also see: Cystitis; Genitourinary system; Stricture of urine; etc.): to help bring temporary relief (up to half an hour or so) from the need to urinate. This technique may be helpful in a situation where facilities are not immediately available, as in driving, etc.

7
24
25
54
69

Urticaria: see Hives and rash (urticaria).

Varicose veins: no G-Jo pressure-point stimulation to be used.

Venereal disease: see Gonorrhea; Sexual organs; etc.

Vertigo (also see: Dizziness; Nausea; Seasickness; Travel sickness; etc.): a sense of dizziness and disorientation caused by a disturbance of the equilibrium and balance mechanisms of the body. Vertigo may be symptomatic of disease or physical and/or mental disturbances.

5
10
24
38
47
65
67
69
77
78
98
99

Vomiting and retching (also see: Nausea; Stomach; etc.): symptomatic of many problems, and not all of them associated with the digestive tract. Dehydration is always a problem with continued loss of fluids; if vomiting is severe, *get medical help immediately.*

6
7
9
10
16
18
23
31
44
48
58
61
71
78
81
86   "morning sickness," early in pregnancy
95

Warm-up control centers (also see: Bioenergy control centers; Frostbite; etc.): to bring a feeling of warmth throughout the body.

29
30
81   to prevent aftereffects of chilling and exposure to wet cold
103

Wasp stings: see Stings, bee and wasp.

Weakness, physical: see Bioenergy control centers; Stamina control centers; etc.

Whiplash (neck injury—also see: Neck; Pain; etc.): a condition that may occur when the neck is snapped suddenly forward or back, as in the event of an automobile accident. *Get medical help immediately.*

1
2   if pain is also in shoulder
5   pain
13
25
116

Wounds (also see: Bruises; specific areas affected such as Arm; Hand; etc.): the rupturing or loss of any body tissues as a result of injury. First, check for arterial and/or venous bleeding; also watch for symptoms of shock. *With any serious wound, get medical help immediately.*

5   pain
21   if body portion is crushed or bruised
22   deep cuts
24   wound where light touch aggravates spasms of the body
26   cuts and lacerations; also, for crushed fingernails
46
57
68   punctures

Wrist (also see: Forearm; Hand).

1   40
4   79
10   116
13
15
18
21

Yawning control center (also see: Respiratory system; etc.): Yawning may be a signal to begin breathing properly or more deeply.

1

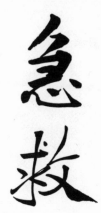

PART III

illustrated points
and their locations

G-Jo Point No. 1 *

One and one-half thumbs above the most prominent crease of the wrist, in line with the thumbnail. A difficult point to find, but made easier by linking the hands as shown in the illustration; the point is found beneath the index finger, which lies along the top of the wrist, deep in a small hollow.

TYPE 1

Chest, plus no. 13
Colds and influenza
Cough
Eye
Face
Head
Headache
Laryngitis
Migraine
Nasal congestion (catarrh)
Neck
Nosebleed (epistaxis)
Respiratory system
Shoulder
Sinusitis
Sore throat
Styes
Throat
Wrist

TYPE 2

Asthma
Bronchitis
Colitis
Concussion
Conjunctivitis
Gall bladder
Heart
Hiccough (hiccup) control center
Lumbago
Lungs
Memory control center
Pain control center
Pleurisy, plus no. 13
Pneumonia, plus no. 13
Whiplash (neck injury)
Yawn control center

G-Jo Point No. 2 *

On the extreme end of the outer crease of the elbow. Bend your arm tightly and place a finger on the end of the crease; keep your finger in place. Open the arm and stimulate the point on your relaxed arm.

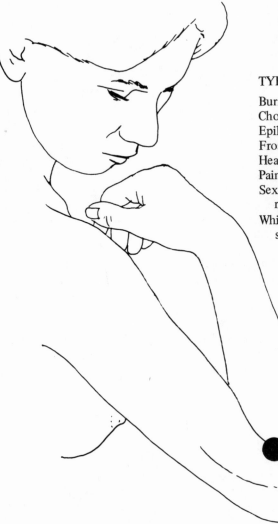

TYPE 1

Acne, plus no. 13
Allergies, plus no. 27 and/or no. 28
Arm
Blisters
Boils
Colds and influenza
Elbow
Eye
Face, plus no. 13
Forearm
Heat rash (miliaria)
Hives and rash (urticaria)
Impetigo and eczema
Itching; itchy skin
Neck
Poison ivy, oak and sumac
Shoulder
Skin
Stomach
Styes

TYPE 2

Burns, especially to help heal skin
Cholera
Epilepsy
Frostbite, plus no. 27 and no. 28
Head injuries, plus no. 21
Pain control center, especially joints
Sexual organs, especially uterus and ovaries
Whiplash (neck injury), especially when shoulder is affected

G-Jo Point No. 3 *

In the center of the crease at the rear of
the knee, between the two ligaments. *Do
not use this point if you have varicose
veins.*

This point not for Type 1 use.

TYPE 2

Abdominal pain
Back, lower, plus no. 5
Bladder
Hypertension (high blood pressure), plus
    no. 69
Impetigo and exzema
Itching; itchy skin
Knee
Leg
Lumbago
Nausea
Nosebleed (epistaxis)
Pain control center (lower back)
Seasickness
Sciatica
Skin problems
Sweating control center
Thigh
Tonsilitis
Travel sickness

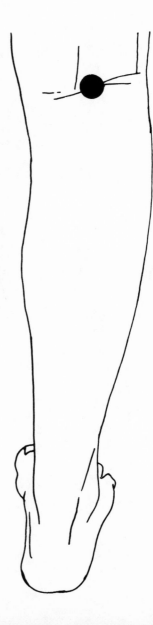

G-Jo Point No. 4 **

The width of two thumbs above the most prominent crease of the *upper* wrist, in line with the middle finger.

TYPE 1

Alcohol problems, plus 37
Anxiety
Arm
Bursitis
Cheeks
Chest
Colds and influenza
Cough
Depression
Ear
Elbow
Facial neuralgia
Hand
Head
Headache
Nervousness
Poison ivy, oak and sumac
Relaxation
Sciatica
Shoulder
Skin
Sore throat
Stress and tension
Wrist

TYPE 2

Cholera
Fear control center
Fever control center
Heart
Heart attack, heart failure
Hemorrhage (severe); bright, red blood; plus no. 43, used alternatingly until bleeding stops
Hypertension (high blood pressure)
Hypoglycemia; plus no. 37
Infantile paralysis, temporary
Mumps
Pain control center (chest and ribs)
Pleurisy
Temper control center
Tonsilitis
Ulcers, intestinal

G-Jo Point No. 5 **

In the hollow (or valley) behind the crown of the *outer* ankle.

TYPE 1

Back, especially lower
Buttocks
Cramps, intestinal and internal (colic)
Coccyx
Face
Foot
Headache
Hemorrhoids
Hip
Impetigo and eczema
Leg
Neuralgia
Rectum
Relaxation
Sprains, muscular
Strains, muscular
Stress and tension
Toothache

TYPE 2

Back, plus no. 3
Burns
Childbirth
Convulsions, especially in children
Foot, plus no. 3
Leg, plus no. 3
Lumbago
Pain control center (general pain)
Sciatica, plus no. 3
Testicles
Vertigo

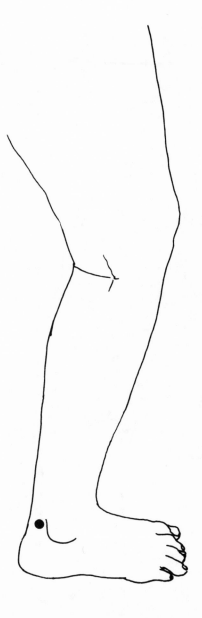

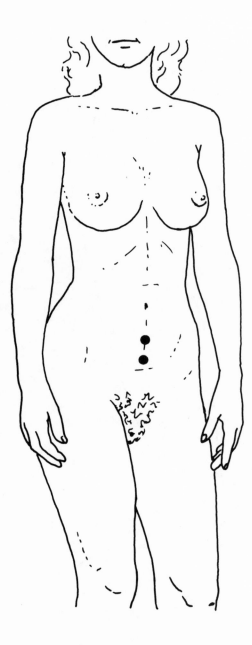

G-Jo Point No. 6

The width of one hand below, and in line with, the navel. Another point is found the width of one to two thumbs directly beneath that point, which may have similar effects.

TYPE 1

Constipation
Diarrhea
Indigestion
Insomnia
Menstruation
Vomiting

TYPE 2

Bioenergy control center
Cholera
Cystitis
Diabetes (diabetes mellitus)
Drowning
Genitourinary system
Hiccup (hiccough) control center
Hypertension (high blood pressure)
Prostate
Sexual organs

TYPE 1

Abdomen, lower, and upper; plus no. 9
Back, lower, plus no. 9
Colon
Constipation
Cramps, intestinal and internal (colic)
Depression
Diarrhea, plus no. 9
Flatulence, plus no. 9
Foot
Gastrointestinal system, plus no. 9 and/or
    no. 13
Genitourinary system
Hangover
Hip, plus no. 9
Impetigo and eczema
Indigestion, plus no. 9
Leg
Lumbago
Menstruation, plus no. 27
Nausea
Pain in testicles and lower back together;
    also in lower part of body
Relaxation
Sciatica, plus no. 9
Seasickness
Stomach, plus no. 9
Travel sickness
Vomiting and retching, plus no. 9

TYPE 2

Childbirth, plus no. 13
Colitis
Cystitis
Diabetes (diabetes mellitus)
Dysentery
Edema
Gall bladder
Hernia, plus no. 9
Hunger control center
Pain control center (lower body)
Prostate
Sexual organs, internal and external
Small intestines
Smoking control center
Spleen, including pancreas
Testicles, plus no. 9
Ulcers, intestinal
Ulcers, peptic
Urinary control center

G-Jo Point No. 7 **

The width of one hand above the crown of the *inner* ankle, just behind the bone (tibia, "shin bone") on the front of the leg.

G-Jo Point No. 8 *

Midway between the anus and the sex organ, atop the crease-like tissue (perineum). This is a seldom-used point, but when stimulated, its effects can be dramatic in cases where life has apparently just ceased.

This point not for Type 1 use.

TYPE 2

Asphyxia (suffocation)*
Bioenergy control center
Cardiac arrest*
Choking, when victim is breathing again*
Concussion, if death seems near
Constipation
Drowning *
Electric shock (electrocution)
Hemorrhoids
Menstrual problems
Prostate
Sexual organs, internal and external
Suffocation*

*This point does not replace the standard Western emergency and first-aid methods.

TYPE 1

Abdomen, lower and upper, plus no. 7
Back, lower
Bladder, urinary
Colds and influenza
Colic
Colon
Constipation
Cough
Depression (massage briskly downward)
Diarrhea, plus no. 7 and/or no. 95
Eye
Fatigue
Flatulence, plus no. 7
Foot
Gastrointestinal system, plus no. 7 and/or
    no. 13
Hangover
Head
Headache
Heat rash (miliaria)
Hip, plus no. 7
Indigestion, plus no. 7
Itching; itchy skin
Knee
Leg
Lumbago
Nausea
Sciatica, plus no. 7
Seasickness
Stomach
Travel sickness
Vomiting and retching, plus no. 7 and/or
    no. 95

TYPE 2

Bioenergy control center
Cholera
Colitis
Diabetes (diabetes mellitus)
Dysentery
Edema
Fear control center, terror and palpita-
    tions
Gall bladder
Hernia, plus no. 7
Hunger control center
Mental problems, temporary
Pain control center (middle and lower body)
Pneumonia

Prostate
Sexual organs, internal and external
Small intestines
Smoking control center
Spleen and pancreas
Tachycardia
Testicles, plus no. 7
Ulcers, intestinal
Ulcers, peptic

*This point is often used alone or in conjunc-
tion with other points for any problem between
the upper abdomen and the toes.

G-Jo Point No. 9 **

The width of one hand below the bottom
of the kneecap; then the width of one
thumb toward the *outside* of the leg
(direction of the small toe). Found in the
trough or valley just away from the most
prominent bone (tibia, "shin bone").*

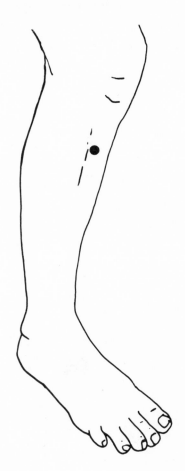

G-Jo Point No. 10 **

The width of two thumbs above the most prominent crease on the *inner* wrist, in line with the middle finger.

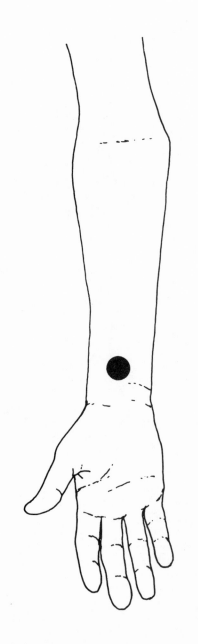

TYPE 1

Abdominal pains
Anxiety
Arm
Armpit, especially if swollen and painful
Breasts
Chest
Cough
Diarrhea
Elbow
Finger
Forearm
Head
Headache
Heartburn
Insomnia
Menstruation
Nervousness
Relaxation
Respiratory system
Seasickness
Shoulder
Stomach
Travel sickness
Vomiting and retching
Wrist

TYPE 2

Angina pectoris
Apoplexy (stroke)
Dizziness
Drowning
Dysentery
Dyspnea
Epileptic seizure
Heart
Heart attack, heart failure
Hiccoughs (hiccups) control center
Jaundice
Memory control center
Pain control center (arm, armpit, shoul-
    der)
Shock
Smoking control center
Sunstroke
Vertigo

G-Jo Point No. 11

In the hollow, but more toward the *outside* (direction of the thumb) of the inner elbow crease.

TYPE 1

Allergies
Cough
Elbow
Laryngitis
Respiratory system
Shoulder
Sore throat
Throat

TYPE 2

Asthma
Bronchitis
Bursitis
Diabetes (diabetes mellitus)
Hemorrhage
Hyperventilation
Lumbago
Pneumonia
Smoking control center
Sneezing control center

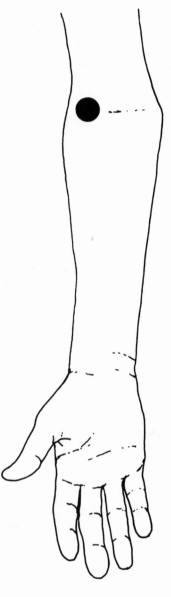

G-Jo Point No. 12 *

Between the nail and the first joint of the thumb, just behind the nail on the side farthest from the other fingers.

TYPE 1

Forearm
Hand
Head
Headache
Laryngitis
Nasal congestion (catarrh)
Respiratory system
Sinusitis
Sore throat
Throat

TYPE 2

Choking*
Convulsions (bright, red face; wild staring, dry eyes)
Drowning*
Fever control center
Meningitis
Sunstroke (mild)
Syncope (fainting)
Tonsilitis
Unconsciousness (face bright red)

*This point does not replace standard Western emergency and first-aid methods.

G-Jo Point No. 13 **

In the webbing between the thumb and forefinger; squeeze the two together and place a finger atop the mound that is formed. Keep your finger on the mound and relax your hand; then begin the stimulation.*

TYPE 1

Acne, plus no. 2
Bursitis
Cheeks
Chest
Colds and influenza
Colic
Colon
Depression
Ear
Elbow
Eye
Face
Facial neuralgia
Foot
Forearm
Gastrointestinal system, plus no. 7 and/or
   no. 9
Gingivitis (bleeding gums)
Hand
Head
Headache
Heat rash (miliaria)
Laryngitis
Lip
Lumbago
Migraine
Mouth
Nasal congestion (catarrh)
Neck
Nervousness, plus no. 17
Neuralgia
Nosebleed (epistaxis)
Relaxation
Respiratory system
Sedation, plus no. 17
Shoulder
Sinusitis
Sore throat
Stress and tension
Throat
Toothache (lower jaw)
Tongue
Wrist

TYPE 2

Asthma
Childbirth, plus no. 7
Concussion
Conjunctivitis
Dislocated bone (for pain)
Gall bladder
Heart
Heart attack, heart failure
Hemorrhage
Mumps
Pain control center (upper body)
Pleurisy, plus no. 1
Pneumonia, plus no. 1
Poisoning; vomiting and retching, face
   pale and blue; cold sweat; plus no. 77
   each half hour until improvement
Sunstroke
Sweating, plus no. 72
Tonsilitis
Whiplash (neck injury)

*Note: this point is often used for any problem from the chest upwards.

G-Jo Point No. 14

The width of one hand and two thumbs below the bottom of the kneecap; then the width of one thumb to the outside of the front bone (tibia, "shin bone"), direction of the small toe. This point is slightly below point no. 9.

TYPE 1

Abdomen, lower
Menstruation

TYPE 2

Appendicitis, acute

G-Jo Point No. 15 *

On the crease of the *inner* wrist, in line
with the smallest finger.

This point not for Type 1 use.

TYPE 2

Angina pectoris
Anxiety
Bedwetting
Dental work, before drilling or extraction
Depression
Electric shock (electrocution), when
    there is restlessness
Fainting, from fear or anxiety
Fear control center, restlessness
Head, headaches
Heart
Heart attack, heart failure, plus no. 46 or
    no. 77
Heartburn
Hysteria
Insomnia, plus no. 46
Migraine
Nervousness
Relaxation
Restlessness
Shock, plus no. 18
Stage fright
Stress and tension
Tachycardia
Temper control center
Wrist

Avoid deep stimulation on this point.

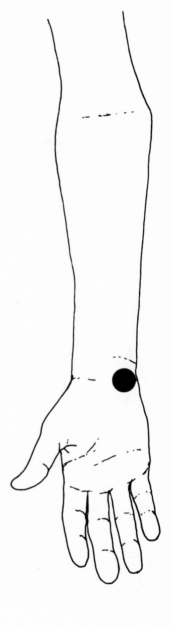

G-Jo Point No. 16

Between the nail and the first joint of the middle finger, closer to the nail, on the side toward the thumb.

TYPE 1

Anxiety
Dental work, before drilling, extraction, etc.
Diarrhea
Menstrual cramps
Vomiting

TYPE 2

Dysentery
Fear control center
Fever (without sweating) control center
Hypertension (high blood pressure)
Hypotension (low blood pressure)
Mental depression, temporary
Restlessness

G-Jo Point No. 17

The width of two thumbs above the separation between the biggest and second toes, top side of the foot.

TYPE 1

Cramps, muscular, plus no. 35; nocturnal leg cramps
Eye
Foot
Headaches
Migraine
Nervousness
Relaxation
Sedation, plus no. 13
Spasms, muscular, plus no. 35

TYPE 2

Asphyxia (suffocation), when face is blue (cyanotic)
Cholera
Genitourinary system
Jaundice
Liver
Poisoning, carbon monoxide
Stricture of urine, plus no. 35
Temper control center

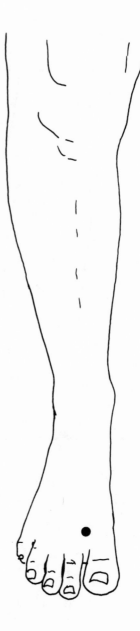

G-Jo Point No. 18 *

On the crease of the *inner* wrist in line with the thumb.

TYPE 1

Arm
Armpit, especially if swollen and painful
Cough, plus no. 107
Eye
Forearm
Hand, especially the thumb
Insomnia
Migraine
Nausea
Throat
Vomiting
Wrist

TYPE 2

Asphyxia (suffocation), face is pale
Asthma
Claustrophilia
Claustrophobia
Concussion, death seems near
Conjunctivitis
Dyspnea (difficult, labored breathing)
Electric shock (electrocution), victim is
    livid like a corpse, unconscious or
    nearly so
Exhaustion and collapse
Poisoning, carbon monoxide
Poisoning, food, if severe, plus no. 53
Shock, plus no. 18, if severe add no. 21
Thirst control center
Unconsciousness, from head injury, when
    there is breathing and no convulsion

G-Jo Point No. 19

The width of one or two thumbs to either side of the spine, on an imaginary line drawn approximately between the mid-forearms (just below the lowest lumbar vertebra).

TYPE 1

Coccyx

TYPE 2

Apoplexy (stroke)
Concussion, if blood is oozing from ears and/or mouth, plus no. 20, *right foot only* and followed in ten minutes by no. 21
Cystitis
Diabetes (diabetes mellitus)
Genital problems
Gonorrhea
Hemorrhage (dark, venous blood)
Lumbago
Prostate
Sciatica
Sexual organs
Small intestines
Snakebite; immediate, deep pressure for one minute; then as necessary

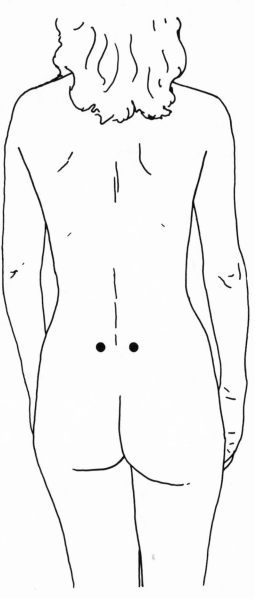

G-Jo Point No. 20

Between the crown of the *inner* ankle and the tip of the heel. The spot that is most pressure-sensitive may be relatively large, compared to other G-Jo points.

TYPE 1

Cough, plus no. 65
Earache
Genitourinary system
Hearing difficulties
Mouth, plus no. 65
Throat, plus no. 65

TYPE 2

Bites, insect and animal
Breath control center
Diabetes (diabetes mellitus)
Gonorrhea
Hemorrhage, plus no. 103, followed in
    ten minutes by no. 21
Kidneys
Malaria
Prostate
Shortness of breath, plus no. 65
Uterus

Right foot only
Bites (and stings), insect; skin is red,
    swollen and waxy-looking
Bites, spider; skin is red, swollen and
    waxy-looking
Frostbite; skin is red, shiny
Stings, bee and wasp, plus no. 25
Stings, scorpion; skin is red, swollen and
    waxy-looking

Left foot only
Apoplexy (stroke)
Concussion; blood oozing from ears and/
    or mouth; plus no. 19, followed in ten
    minutes by no. 21
Frostbite; skin is blue
Hemorrhage; dark, venous blood
Snakebite; immediate, deep pressure for
    one minute, then as necessary
Unconsciousness; breathing is present and
    no convulsions

G-Jo Point No. 21

At the point of the shoulders. Raise your arm slightly above the level of your shoulder and place a finger in the for- wardmost dimple; then, keeping your finger in the dimple, lower your arm and begin stimulation.

TYPE 1

Arm, alone or plus no. 2
Bruises, if skin is not broken, plus no.
   103
Fatigue, physical
Head, plus no. 2
Neck, plus no. 2
Shoulders, plus no. 2
Wrist

TYPE 2

Apoplexy (stroke)
Concussion
Electric shock (electrocution); severe
   cases; skin is pale, cold, clammy
Exhaustion (physical)
Head injuries, plus no. 2
Hemorrhage; dark, venous blood
Hypertension
Shock; plus no. 18, if severe
Unconsciousness; from head injury,
   breathing present and no convulsions
Wounds, if body portion crushed or bruised

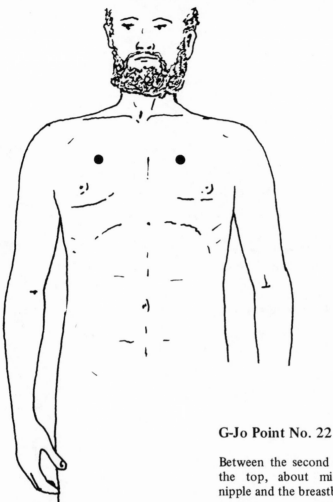

G-Jo Point No. 22

Between the second and third ribs from the top, about midway between the nipple and the breastbone (sternum).

This point has no Type 1 use.

TYPE 2

Bites, animal and human
Bites, insect; if skin is cold
Bites, spider; if skin is cold
Stings, bee and wasp; if skin is cold
Stings, scorpion; if skin is cold
Tetanus (lockjaw); to help prevent tetanus, this point should be used immediately after the injury occurs, *left side only*
Wounds, punctures and deep cuts

G-Jo Point No. 23

On the spine, in the valley between the lowest cervical and the highest dorsal vertebrae; on an imaginary line drawn between the tips of the shoulders.

TYPE 1

Colds and influenza
Cough, especially a hacking cough
Hives and rash (urticaria)
Neck
Nosebleed (epistaxis)
Vomiting

TYPE 2

Cholera
Jaundice
Paralysis, temporary
Pleurisy, plus no. 10

G-Jo Point No. 24

Just behind the bony prominence located to the rear of the smallest toe, on the outside edge of the foot.

TYPE 1

Face; facial pain
Genitourinary system
Jaw, lower and upper
Neuralgia
Rectum
Sunburn
Toothache
Vertigo

TYPE 2

Bites, insect (including fleas and mosquitoes); skin is inflamed, hot and red
Bites, spider; skin is inflamed, hot and red
Bladder
Burns and scalds
Colitis
Cystitis
Lumbago
Pain control center, especially face
Poisoning by mouth, burning sensation in mouth; throat feels on fire; swallowing only with difficulty; face pale and wretched
Prostate
Sciatica
Stings, bee and wasp
Sting, scorpion; skin is inflamed, hot and red
Urinary control center; to ease the need to urinate for up to half an hour
Wounds, when light touch triggers spasms

G-Jo Point No. 25

On the outside edge of the foot, just
ahead of the bony prominence (direction
of toes) found midway between the toes
and the ankle.

TYPE 1

Bladder, urinary
Neck

TYPE 2

Bites, spider
Stings, bee and wasp, especially if the
    throat is swollen, puffy, fiery and/or
    red; plus no. 20
Urinary control center; to ease the need
    to urinate for up to half an hour
Whiplash (neck injury)

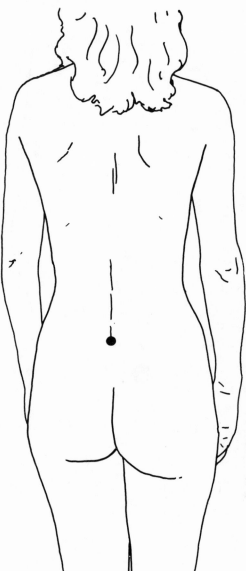

G-Jo Point No. 26

On the spine at the fifth lumbar vertebra, on an imaginary line drawn between the mid-forearms.

TYPE 1

Dental work; every two hours after extraction or painful dental work

TYPE 2

Bioenergy control center
Bruises, skin is broken, plus no. 103
Concussion, if caused by spinal injury
Fingernails, torn or crushed
Fracture, for relief of pain
Unconsciousness; from spinal injury, breathing is present and *no* convulsions
Wounds, if body portion is cut or lacerated

G-Jo Point No. 27

The width of two thumbs above the top of the kneecap, in the inner thigh, approximately in line with the crown of the inner ankle.

TYPE 1

Acne
Allergies, plus no. 2 and/or no. 28
Blisters
Boils
Menstruation, plus no. 7
Poison ivy, oak and sumac
Skin
Styes

TYPE 2

Burns; to help heal, plus no. 2 and/or no. 20
Frostbite, plus no. 2 and no. 28

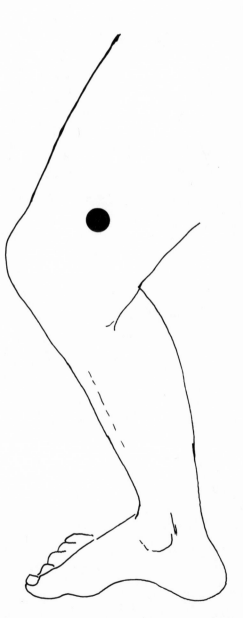

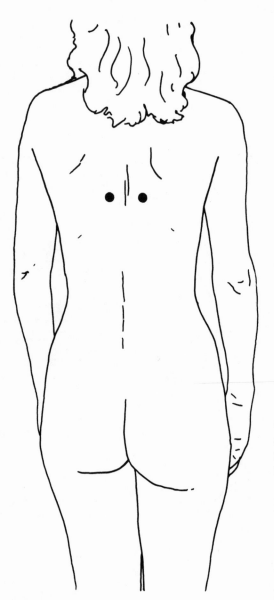

G-Jo Point No. 28

The width of one thumb to either side of the spine, along an imaginary line drawn between the bottoms of the shoulder blades.

TYPE 1

Acne
Allergies, plus no. 2 and/or no. 27
Bladder, urinary
Blisters
Boils
Poison ivy, oak and sumac
Skin
Styes

TYPE 2

Burns, to help heal skin
Cerebral hemorrhage
Diabetes (diabetes mellitus)
Frostbite, plus no. 2 and no. 27

G-Jo Point No. 29

On the top of the shoulder, midway
between the tip of the shoulder and the
neck.

TYPE 1

Arm
Back, upper
Boils
Neck
Shoulder

TYPE 2

Breasts
Frostbite, also, to help prevent frostbite
Pain control center (upper back)
Warm-up control center; to help create a
    feeling of warmth, and to increase
    circulation

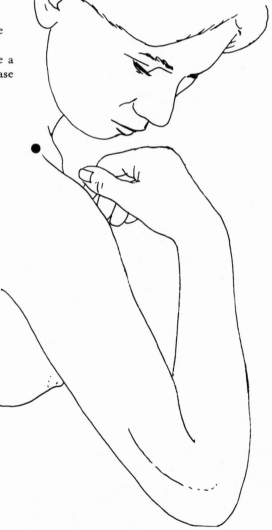

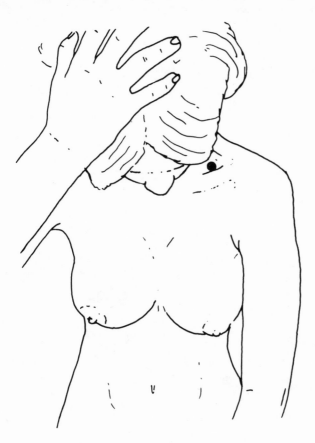

G-Jo Point No. 30

Hunch shoulders forward as far as possible; two hollows will be formed just behind the collarbone (clavicle). Place one or several fingers in each hollow (deepest part), and relax the shoulders. Keep your finger(s) in the area and begin the stimulation.

This point has no Type 1 use.

TYPE 2

Edema
Frostbite, and to help prevent frostbite
Warm-up control center; to help create a
    feeling of warmth, and to increase
    circulation

G-Jo Point No. 31

Immediately below the bottom of the breastbone (sternum) where the most sensitive area is found (xiphoid process), in line with the navel.

TYPE 1

Colic
Indigestion
Seasickness
Travel sickness
Vomiting and retching

TYPE 2

Bioenergy control center
Heart
Hiccough (hiccups) control center
Mental disturbances, temporary
Smoking control center
Temper control center

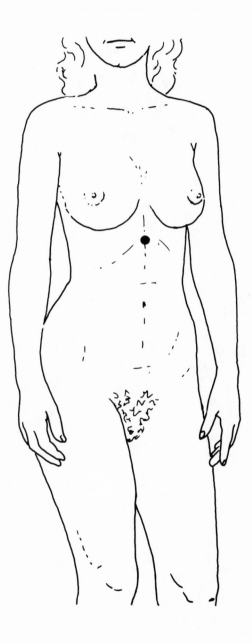

G-Jo Point No. 32

On the spine, between the fourth and fifth dorsal vertebrae, in line with the middle of the shoulder blades.

TYPE 1

Nervousness (in children); massage downwards
Nosebleed (epistaxis)

TYPE 2

Bioenergy control center
Bites, animal and insect
Convulsions; violent, epileptic
Epileptic seizures
Mental disturbances (suicidal actions)
Rabid animal bites; stimulate several times each hour
Unconsciousness; violent, epileptic

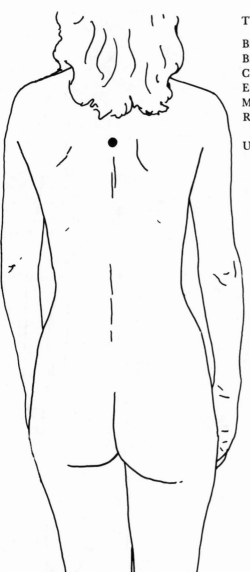

G-Jo Point No. 33

On the outer edge of the hand, directly behind the rearmost knuckle of the littlest finger.

TYPE 1

Eye
Forearm

TYPE 2

Convulsions; violent, epileptic
Intestinal cramps and spasms,
    violent; eyes wet
Malaria
Mumps
Unconsciousness; violent, epileptic

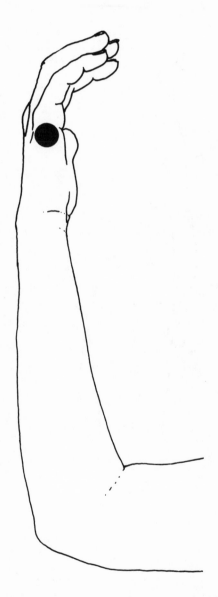

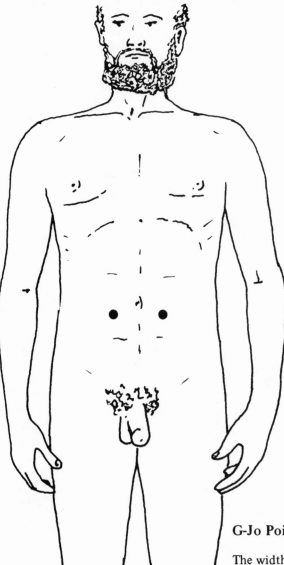

G-Jo Point No. 34

The width of one hand either side of, and
the width of one thumb below the navel.

TYPE 1

Constipation

TYPE 2

Convulsions; hysterical, face is pale
Fainting; with hysterical symptoms
Hysteria
Unconsciousness, with face pale and hysteria

G-Jo Point No. 35

Slightly behind (direction of the rear of the foot, topside) the separation between the biggest and the second toes.

TYPE 1

Cramps, muscular; plus no. 17
Impetigo and exzema
Insomnia
Neck
Nervousness
Shoulder
Spasms, muscular, plus no. 17

TYPE 2

Beriberi
Carbuncles
Convulsions and fits, especially in children
Fear control center
Fear in children
Genitourinary system
Gout
Liver
Menstruation; excessive menses
Stricture of urine
Temper control center

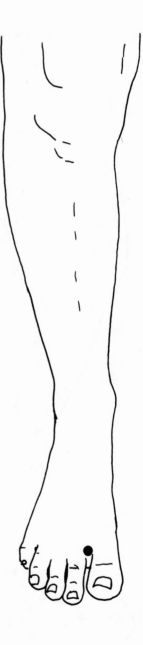

G-Jo Point No. 36

The width of one hand, plus the width of two thumbs, above the crown of the *inner* ankle, just to the rear of the front bone (tibia, "shin bone").

TYPE 1

Abdomen, lower
Abdomen, upper

TYPE 2

Genitourinary system
Stricture of urine, plus no 17 and/or
   no. 35

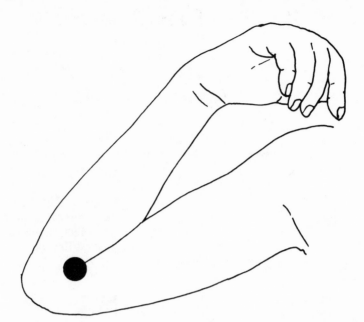

G-Jo Point No. 37

At the extreme end of the *inner* crease of the elbow. Bend the arm tightly and place a finger or thumb at the extreme inner edge of the elbow crease formed. Relax your arm and begin the stimulation.

This point not for Type 1 use.

TYPE 2

Alcohol problems, plus 4
Bursitis
Depression
Dizziness
Exhaustion (mental)
Fatigue (light, brisk upward stimulation
Fear control center, terror and palpitations
Epilepsy
Forearm
Hypoglycemia, plus 4
Stress and tension
Tachycardia
Temper control center
Toothache

* Avoid deep stimulation on this point.

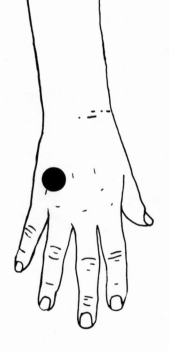

G-Jo Point No. 38

On the top of the hand, midway between the rearmost knuckles and the wrist; in the valley between the third and the smallest fingers.

TYPE 1

Back
Eye
Facial neuralgia
Hand
Headache
Sciatica

TYPE 2

Conjunctivitis
Dizziness
Exhaustion (physical)
Lumbago
Malaria
Pain control center (middle back)
Tonsilitis
Vertigo

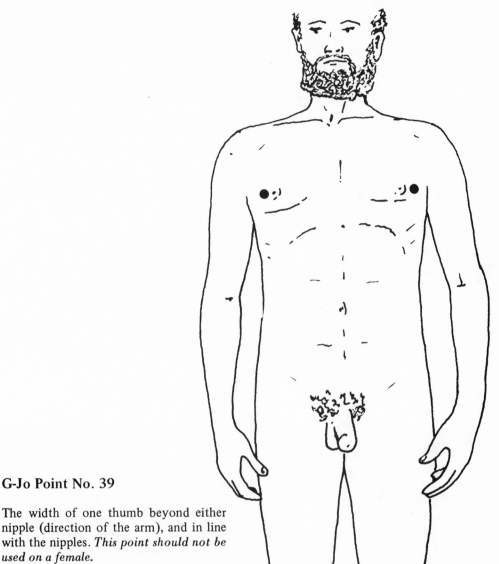

G-Jo Point No. 39

The width of one thumb beyond either
nipple (direction of the arm), and in line
with the nipples. *This point should not be
used on a female.*

TYPE 1

Armpit, especially if swollen and painful
Forearm

TYPE 2

Fainting, from heart failure
Heart atack, heart failure

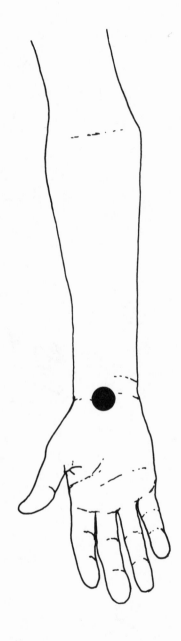

G-Jo Point No. 40

On the most prominent crease of the *inner* wrist, in line with the middle finger.

TYPE 1

Corns, bunions
Hand
Impetigo and eczema
Insomnia
Skin
Wrist

TYPE 2

Fainting, from heart failure
Heart
Heart attack, heart failure
Hypertension (high blood pressure)
Pain control center (neuralgia between
    the ribs)

G-Jo Point No. 41

Near the "ball-joint" of the hips; squeeze the buttocks together tightly. Place a finger in the depression formed at the hip; relax the buttocks and begin the stimulation.

TYPE 1

Anxiety
Buttocks
Frigidity
Hip
Impotence
Sprains, muscular
Sexual organs
Thigh

TYPE 2

Cystitis (use deep pressure)
Paralysis, temporary
Sciatica
Ulcers, stomach, duodenal

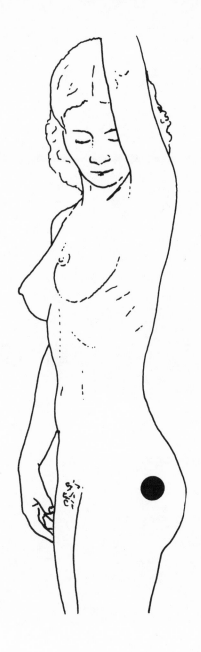

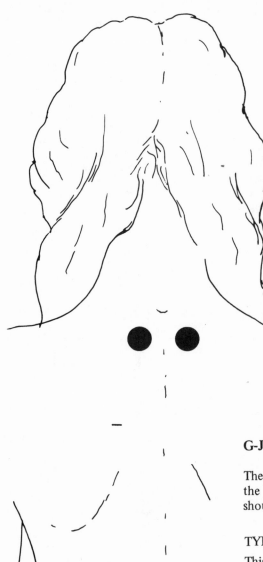

G-Jo Point No. 42

The width of one thumb to either side of the spine, in line with the tips of the shoulders.

TYPE 1

This point has no Type 1 use.

TYPE 2

Bones
Epilepsy
Fear control center, terror and palpitations
Fracture; to help bones knit more rapidly
Sciatica
Tachycardia

G-Jo Point No. 43

On the top of the foot, in the valley between the smallest and fourth toes, midway between the separation between the toes and where the foot joins the leg.

TYPE 1

Neck
Shoulder
Stomach

TYPE 2

Hemorrhage, severe; bright, red blood; use alternatingly with no. 4 until bleeding stops
Temper control center

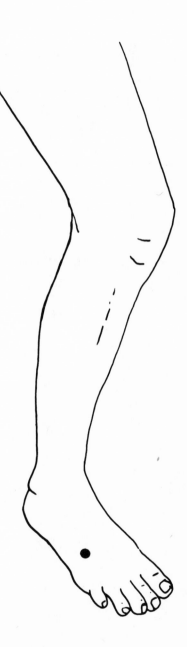

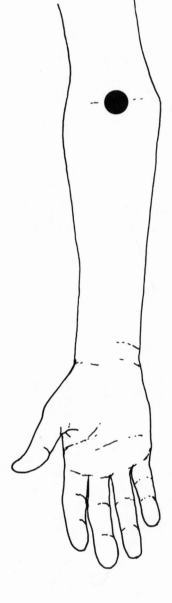

G-Jo Point No. 44

In the deepest hollow of the inner elbow, along the crease, between the two ligaments.

TYPE 1

Arm; pain in upper arm
Cough
Diarrhea
Elbow
Vomiting

TYPE 2

Bronchitis
Cholera
Dysentery
Hemorrhage; bright, red blood; not severe
Measles (after rash has erupted)
Thirst control center

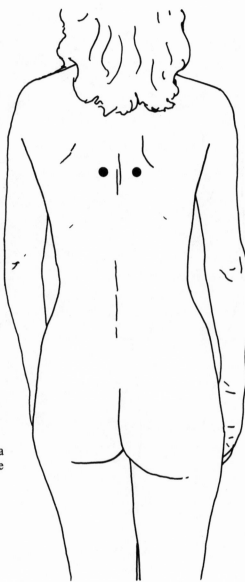

G-Jo Point No. 45

On either side of the spine, just above a line drawn between the bottom of the shoulder blades.

TYPE 1

Anxiety
Ear
Earache
Nervousness, mild or extreme

TYPE 2

Breath control center
Hiccoughs (hiccups) control center; (massage downwards)
Numbness

G-Jo Point No. 46

Just to the rear of the second toenail, on the side closest to the smallest toe.

TYPE 1

Eye
Foot
Hangover
Indigestion
Insomnia, plus no. 15
Sinusitis
Stomach
Toothache (upper jaw)

TYPE 2

Heart, plus no. 15
Heart attack, heart failure, plus no. 15
Tonsilitis
Wounds (light touch triggers spasms) plus
   no. 24 and no. 57

G-Jo Point No. 47

On the spine, in the valley between the first and second dorsal vertebrae; on a line approximately between the tips of the shoulders.

TYPE 1

Back
Neck
Shoulder

TYPE 2

Bioenergy control center
Mental depression, temporary
Mountain sickness (hypoxia)
Pain control center (neck, shoulder, upper back)
Vertigo

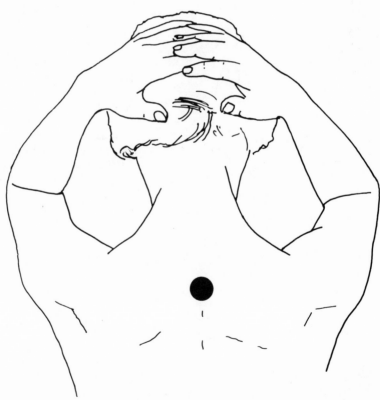

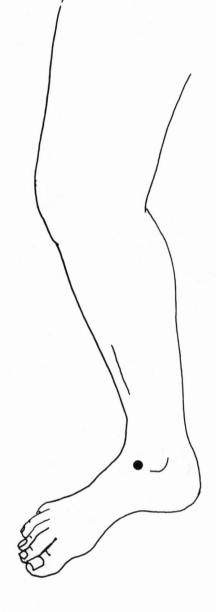

G-Jo Point No. 48

The width of one thumb directly in front of the crown of the *inner* ankle.

TYPE 1

Constipation
Cough
Foot
Vomiting and retching

TYPE 2

Asphyxia (suffocation) plus no. 58
Edema
Gout
Hypertension
Pain control center (testicles, lower back)
    plus no. 7 and no. 58
Spleen, including pancreas
Testicles, crushed or injured; plus no. 58

G-Jo Point No. 49

Just beneath the ear, along the rear of the jawbone.

TYPE 1

Eye
Lumbago
Mouth
Tongue, especially swollen

TYPE 2

Hemorrhage
Intoxication
Pain control center, especially face

G-Jo Point No. 50

The width of one thumb directly in front of the crown of the *outer* ankle, in the valley that is just ahead of the crown.

TYPE 1

Buttocks
Hip
Neck

TYPE 2

Abdominal problems, violent
Conjunctivitis
Hernia
Paralysis, temporary
Poisoning by mouth, violent abdominal
    pains

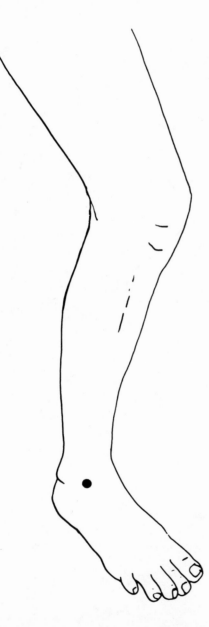

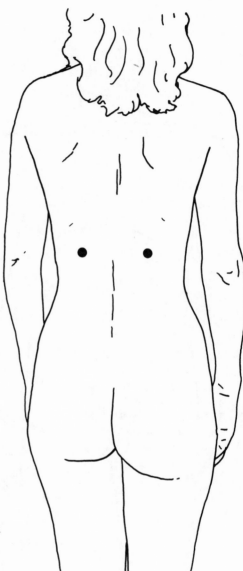

G-Jo Point No. 51

The width of one hand to either side of the spine, on a line drawn between the elbows.

TYPE 1

Back

TYPE 2

Poisoning by mouth; mouth burns, throat feels dry, fiery, hard swallowing; face is pale and wretched.

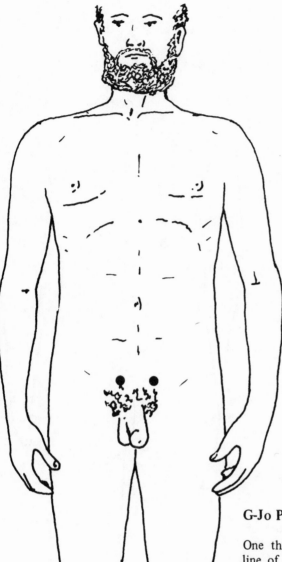

G-Jo Point No. 52

One thumb to either side of the center
line of the front of the body, just at or
slightly above the pubic hair line.

This point has no Type 1 use.

TYPE 2

Poisoning by mouth; mouth burns, throat
   feels fiery, hard swallowing; face is
   pale and wretched.
Sexual organs

G-Jo Point No. 53

On the top of the foot, where the foot meets the leg, in line with the second toe.

TYPE 1

Gingivitis (bleeding gums)
Stomach
Toothache

TYPE 2

Bronchitis
Poisoning, food; restlessness, exhaustion, burning pains, nausea, swollen face; face is pale, cold, sweaty, plus no. 18

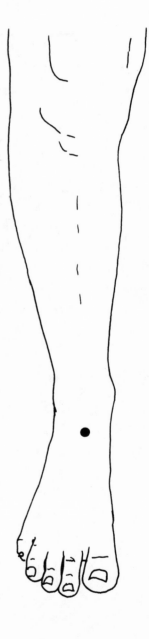

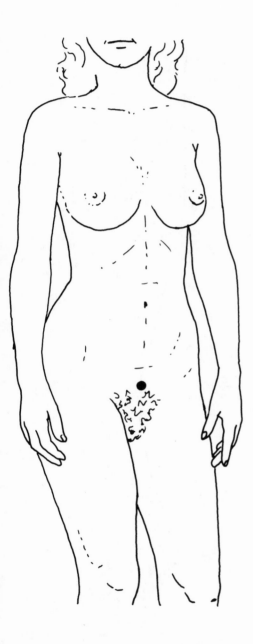

G-Jo Point No. 54

On the front, center line of the body, in line with, or slightly into, the pubic hair line.

TYPE 1

Fatigue
Genitourinary system
Sprains, muscular

TYPE 2

Bladder
Fainting
Sexual organs, internal and external
Urinary control center

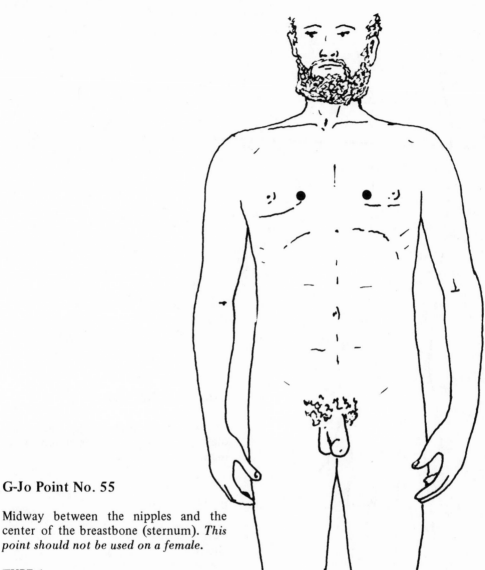

G-Jo Point No. 55

Midway between the nipples and the center of the breastbone (sternum). *This point should not be used on a female.*

TYPE 1

Cough

TYPE 2

Bronchitis
Sunstroke, severe

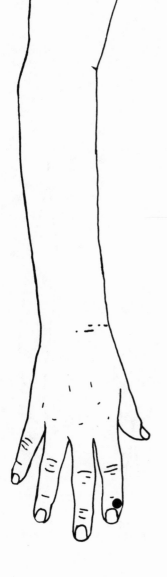

G-Jo Point No. 56

Just behind the corner of the fingernail of the index finger, on the side closest to the thumb.

TYPE 1

Bladder, urinary
Eye
Hearing difficulties
Laryngitis
Jaw, lower
Toothache

TYPE 2

Deafness; sudden, partial
Dental work; while work is in progress

G-Jo Point No. 57

On the *inner* portion of the leg, just below the level of the kneecap, in the concave depression just above the calf; in line with the crown of the *inner* ankle.

TYPE 1

Cramps, muscular
Frigidity
Knee
Spasms, muscular

TYPE 2

Edema
Sciatica
Sexual organs, impotence
Spleen, including pancreas
Wounds, when light touch triggers spasms
    and/or sharp pain; (use left leg only)

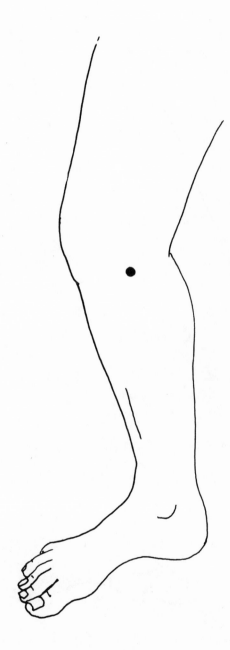

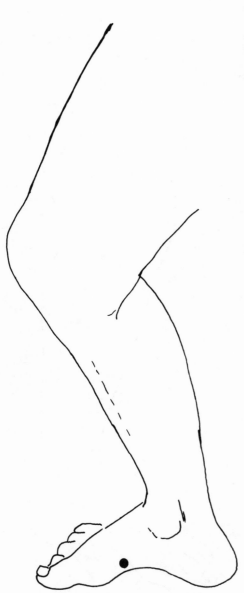

G-Jo Point No. 58

On the *inner* edge of the foot, midway
between the heel and the big toe.

TYPE 1

Back, lower
Foot
Vomiting and retching

TYPE 2

Gout
Pain control center; (testicles, lower
   back) plus no. 7 and no. 48
Pleurisy
Spleen, including pancreas
Suffocation, plus no. 48
Testicles; severe injuries

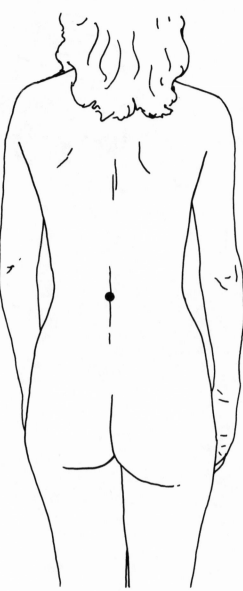

G-Jo Point No. 59

On the spine, atop the third lumbar vertebra, in line with the waist on a "normal-waisted" person.

TYPE 1

Eye
Headache
Insomnia

TYPE 2

Exhaustion, extreme physical and/or
    mental
Pain control center (lower back and lower
    abdomen, together)
Stricture of urine

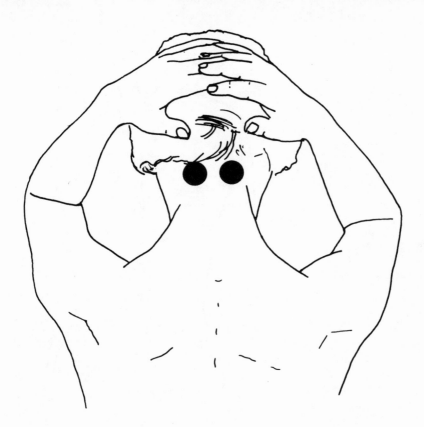

G-Jo Point No. 60

Just beneath the base of the skull, either side of the cervical atlas (where the spine meets the skull).

TYPE 1

Earache
Hearing problems
Nasal congestion (catarrh)
Nosebleed (epistaxis)
Tinnitus

TYPE 2

Fear control center, terror and palpitations
Lightheadedness
Pain control center, especially "writer's cramp"
Tachycardia

G-Jo Point No. 61

The width of one hand above the most prominent crease on the *upper* wrist, in line with the middle finger.

TYPE 1

Arm
Back
Cough
Hand
Impetigo and eczema
Loin area
Shoulder
Vomiting and retching

TYPE 2

Asthma
Cholera
Fever control center
Pain control center (chest, ribs, arm, shoulder, loins)
Pneumonia
Tetanus (lockjaw)

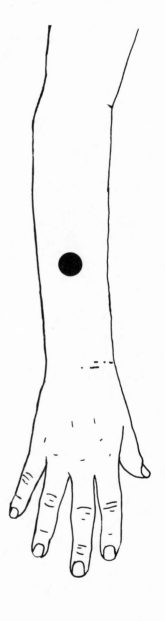

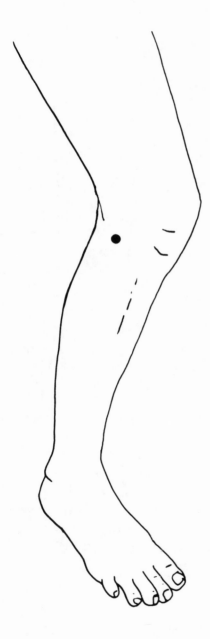

G-Jo Point No. 62

Slightly below the level of the bottom of the kneecap, on the *outer* side of the leg, in the slight depression formed when the knee is completely straight. Forward of a line to the crown of the *outer* ankle.

TYPE 1

Bladder, urinary
Constipation
Cramps, muscular; nocturnal leg cramps
Hip
Knee
Leg
Muscles
Sciatica
Shoulder
Sprains, muscular
Strains, muscular
Stomach
Thigh

TYPE 2

Fear control center, extreme fright
Hernia
Irrationaltiy, temporary
Stamina control center

G-Jo Point No. 63

The width of one hand and one thumb above the crown of the *outer* ankle.

TYPE 1

Buttocks
Hip
Knee

TYPE 2

Goiter
Pain control center
Paralysis, temporary
Sciatica

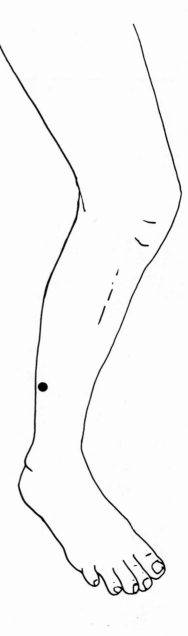

G-Jo Point No. 64

Just behind the corner of the fourth toenail, on the side closest to the smallest toe.

TYPE 1

Cough
Ear
Headache
Hearing difficulties
Insomnia

TYPE 2

Deafness; partial, sudden, temporary
Sleep control center

G-Jo Point No. 65

The width of two hands and one thumb
above the crown of the *outer* ankle; and
nearly in line with, but slightly behind, a
line vertical to the outer ankle.

TYPE 1

Constipation
Cough, plus no. 20
Cramps, muscular; nocturnal leg
    cramps
Hemorrhoids
Mouth, plus no. 20
Rectum
Throat, plus no. 20

TYPE 2

Breath control center
Cystitis
Dizziness
Epileptic seizures
Lumbago
Stamina control center
Vertigo

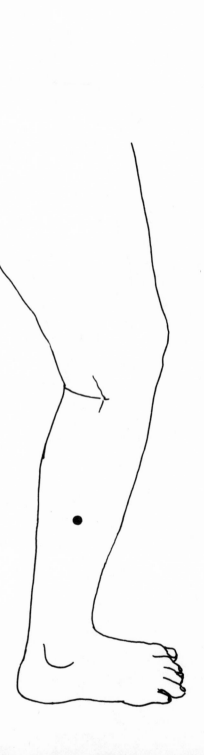

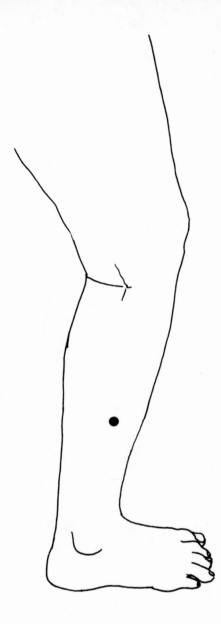

G-Jo Point No. 66

The width of two hands above the crown of the *outer* ankle, and slightly forward of a line vertical to the outer ankle.

TYPE 1

Eye
Migraine

TYPE 2

Conjunctivitis
Eye, plus no. 17
Liver
Temper control center

G-Jo Point No. 67

Where the foot meets the leg, in line with the separation between the second and third toes.

TYPE 1

Constipation
Foot
Gingivitis (bleeding gums)
Headache
Hip
Stomach
Toothache

TYPE 2

Vertigo

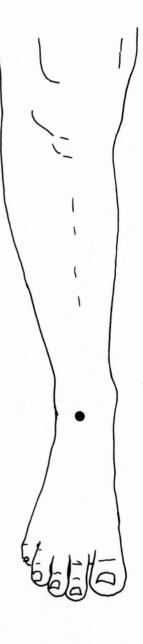

G-Jo Point No. 68

Just behind the nail of the big toe, near the corner on the side closest to the other toes.

TYPE 1

Abdominal pains
Constipation
Foot
Headache

TYPE 2

Fainting (syncope)
Genitourinary system
Gonorrhea
Hernia
Menstruation; excessive flow of menses
Pain control center; (penis, uterus, etc.)
Sleep control center
Spleen, including pancreas
Stricture of urine
Tetanus
Unconsciousness
Wounds, puncture

G-Jo Point No. 69

On the bottom of the foot, in the middle, just behind the ball (most padded forward part).

TYPE 1

Anxiety
Back, lower
Colds and influenza
Foot
Genitourinary system
Head
Headache (top part of head)

TYPE 2

Bioenergy control center
Fear in children
Hypertension (high blood pressure), plus no. 3
Hysteria and panic
Kidneys
Shock: knuckle percussion 12 times
Stricture of urine
Urinary control center
Vertigo

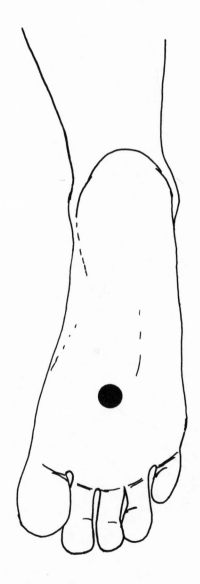

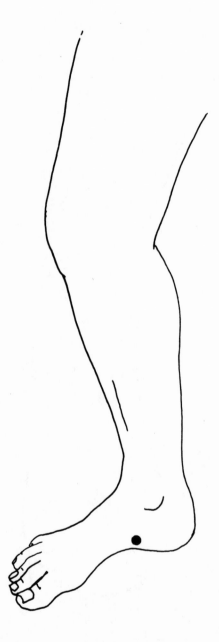

G-Jo Point No. 70

On the *inner* edge of the foot, the width of one hand forward (direction of toes) from the tip of the heel.

TYPE 1

Back, lower
Foot
Sweating at night, during sleep

TYPE 2

Convulsions, especially in children
Cystitis
Sexual organs; internal and external

G-Jo Point No. 71

On a line drawn between the crown of the *inner* ankle and the tip of the heel, the width of two thumbs from the tip of the heel.

TYPE 1

Constipation
Anxiety
Vomiting

TYPE 2

For more serious problems associated with Type 1 symptoms.

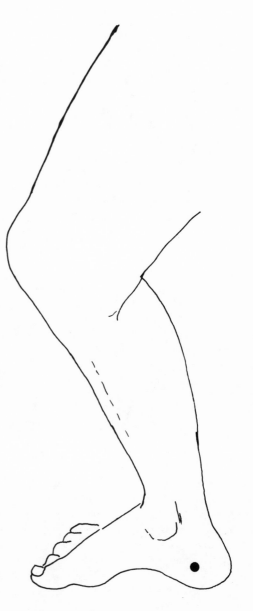

G-Jo Point No. 72

The width of two thumbs above the crown of the *inner* ankle, still on the inner side of the leg, but almost to the rear of the leg.

TYPE 1

Ankle, especially if swollen
Flatulence
Foot
Forearm
Frigidity
Hemorrhoids, bleeding
Shoulder, especially the joint
Toothache

TYPE 2

Diabetes (diabetes mellitus)
Edema
Gonorrhea
Paralysis of the lower limbs, temporary
Prostate
Sweating control center, plus no. 13
Testicles, crushed or injured

G-Jo Point No. 73

On the crease at the rear of the knee, toward the *inner* side of the leg. *Do not use this point if you suffer from varicose veins.*

This point not for Type 1 use.

TYPE 2

Abdomen distended
Heart
Pain control center (genitals, thighs)
Sexual organs, internal and external
Thigh, especially for pain in inner thigh

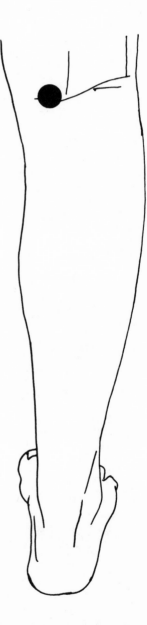

G-Jo Point No. 74

Just behind the separation between the second and third toes.

TYPE 1

Flatulence
Gingivitis (bleeding gums)
Nosebleed (epistaxis)
Toothache (upper jaw)

TYPE 2

Gout

G-Jo Point No. 75

Just behind the outside corner of the nail of the smallest toe (direction away from the other toes). *This point not to be used if you are prone to chronic pain around the eyes.*

TYPE 1

Bladder, urinary
Eye (see precaution above)
Headache
Nasal congestion (catarrh)
Sciatica

TYPE 2

Burns and scalds
Childbirth; to ease delivery
Pain control center
Paralysis, temporary

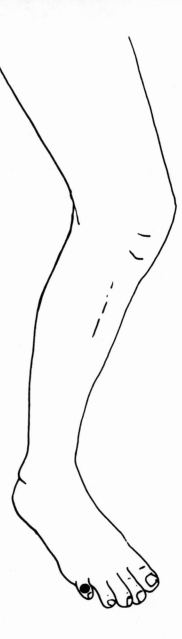

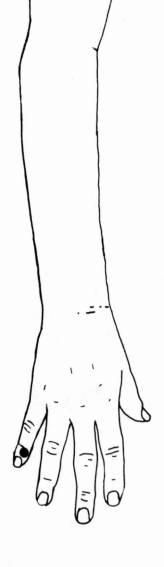

G-Jo Point No. 76

Just behind the inside corner of the nail of the smallest finger (direction toward the other fingers).

This point not for Type 1 use.

TYPE 2

Cardiac arrest
Fatigue (light, brisk upward
    stimulation)
Forearm
Heart attack, heart failure
Heartburn
Mental depression, temporary
Pleurisy

Avoid deep stimulation on this point.

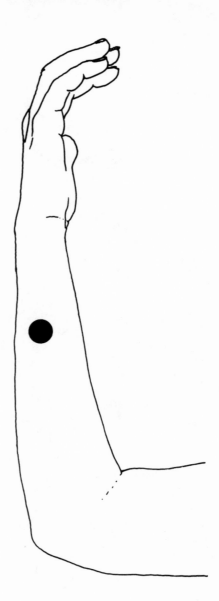

G-Jo Point No. 77

The width of one hand and two thumbs above (direction toward the elbow) the most prominent crease of the wrist, along the bottom edge of the forearm, in line with the smallest finger.

TYPE 1

Forearm
Hand, especially pain in the hand

TYPE 2

Dizziness
Fear control center (apprehension)
Heart, plus no. 15
Pain control center
Poisoning by mouth; vomiting and purg-
    ing present; face is pale, blue and
    covered with cold sweat; plus no. 13 at
    half-hourly intervals
 Vertigo

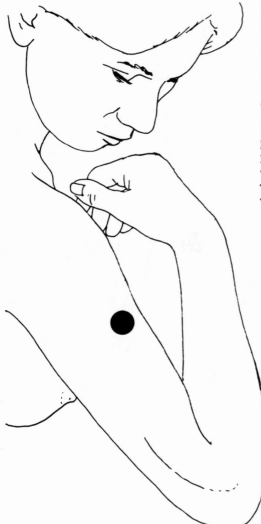

G-Jo Point No. 78

The width of two hands below (direction toward the elbow) the tip of the shoulder, midway between the forward and rearward portion of the upper arm.

TYPE 1

Vomiting

TYPE 2

Bronchitis
Memory control center
Poisoning, carbon monoxide
"Possession by demons"
Thirst control center
Vertigo

G-Jo Point No. 79

The width of one thumb above the most prominent crease of the *inner* wrist, in line with the smallest finger.

This point not for Type 1 use.

TYPE 2

Breath, shortness of
Depression (whisk gently *toward*
    fingers)
Diabetes (diabetes mellitus)
Dizziness
Hand
Hemorrhage
Mental disturbances, temporary
Nasal congestion (catarrh)
Nosebleed (epistaxis)
Pain control center (hand)
Stomach
Tonsilitis
Wrist

*Avoid deep stimulation on this point.

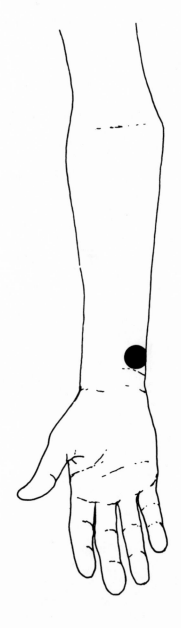

G-Jo Point No. 80A

At the *inner* corner of the eye, very near
and slightly above the tear duct; massage
between the notch you feel above the eye
in the skull opening and the tear duct.

TYPE 1

Eye
Headaches, especially above eyes
Sinusitis

TYPE 2

Conjunctivitis

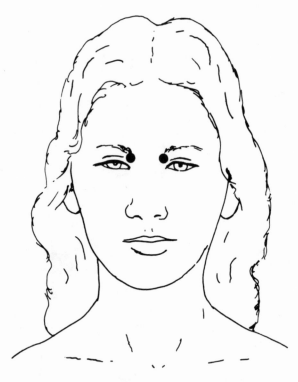

G-Jo Point No. 80B

Just below or within the eyebrow, very near to, but not to be confused with, no. 80A. This point is closer to the center of the eye, just above to just beyond the notch that can be felt in the skull opening (direction of the ears).

TYPE 1

Allergy, hay fever-like symptoms
Back, lower
Eye
Neck
Sinusitis

TYPE 2

Conjunctivitis
Sciatica
Sneezing control center

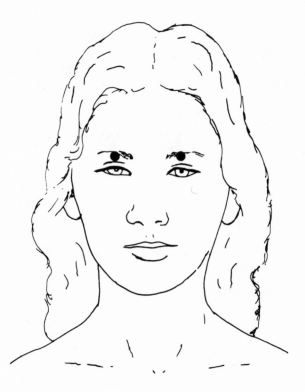

G-Jo Point No. 81

The width of one thumb to either side of
the spine, slightly below a line between
the tips of the shoulders.

TYPE 1

Acne, especially on upper back,
    shoulders
Chilling, to prevent after-effects of being
    chilled or wet
Colds and influenza
Cough
Headache
Nosebleed (epistaxis)
Vomiting and retching

TYPE 2

Asthma
Dizziness
Fear control center, terror and palpitations
Heart
Sexual organs
Sneezing control center
Tachycardia
Warm-up control center

G-Jo Point No. 82

The width of one thumb to either side of the spine, between the fifth and sixth ribs, or along a line between the middle of the shoulder blades.

TYPE 1

Anxiety (nervous, active fear)
Nosebleed (epistaxis
Toothache (molar area)

TYPE 2

Heart
Mountain sickness (hypoxia)
Sunstroke

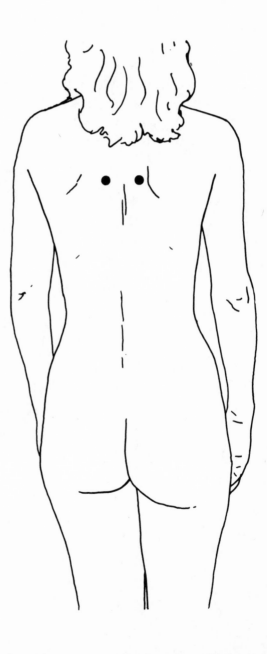

G-Jo Point No. 83

The width of two thumbs to either side
of the spine on, or a little below, on a line
between the elbows.

TYPE 1

Back, upper
Hemorrhoids

TYPE 2

Appendicitis, acute
Edema
Gonorrhea
Hypertension (high blood pressure)
Sciatica

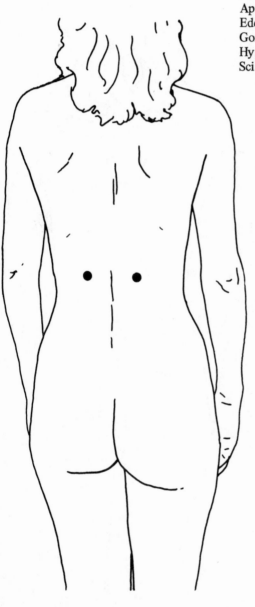

G-Jo Point No. 84

Just below the collarbone (clavicle), in the hollow where the arms join the body.

TYPE 1

Acne
Eyes
Insomnia
Respiratory system
Stomach

TYPE 2

Asthma
Pleurisy and respiratory pain
Pneumonia
Stuttering control center
Tonsilitis

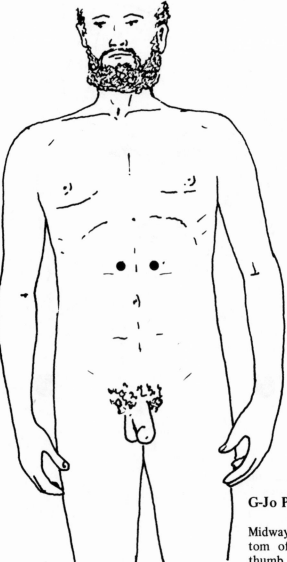

G-Jo Point No. 85

Midway between the navel and the bottom of the ribcage, the width of one thumb to either side of the mid-line.

TYPE 1

Flatulence

TYPE 2

Asthma, and asthmatic breathing
Ulcer, duodenal
Ulcer, peptic

G-Jo Point No. 86

Just below the bottom of the ribcage, the width of one thumb to either side of the mid-line.

TYPE 1

Vomiting, early pregnancy ("Morning Sickness")

TYPE 2

Bronchitis
Jaundice
Ulcer, duodenal
Ulcer, peptic

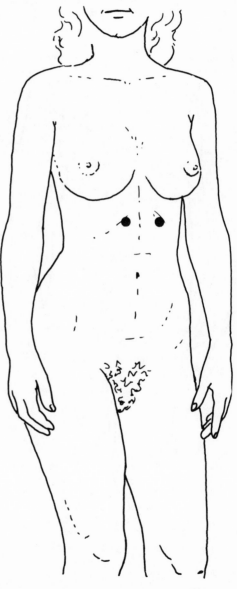

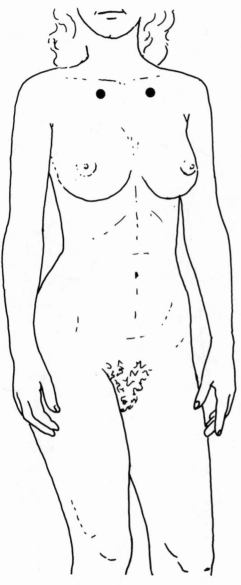

G-Jo Point No. 87

Just below the collarbone (clavicle), in line with the outside edges of the neck, in the hollows below the collarbone.

TYPE 1

Headache, especially from mental strain
Premenstrual discomfort and tension
Tongue, especially if painful

TYPE 2

Asthma
Pain control center

G-Jo Point No. 88

The width of one hand and one thumb above the most prominent crease on the *inner* wrist, in line with the middle finger.

TYPE 1

Arm
Armpit, especially if swollen and painful
Ear
Head
Nightmares, especially in children

TYPE 2

Choking (object stuck in throat) *
Cholera
Fear control center, fear in children
Malaria
Pain control center (ear)

*This point does not replace the standard Western emergency and first-aid methods.

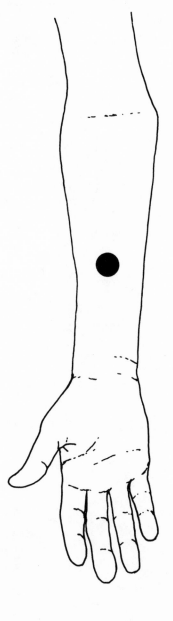

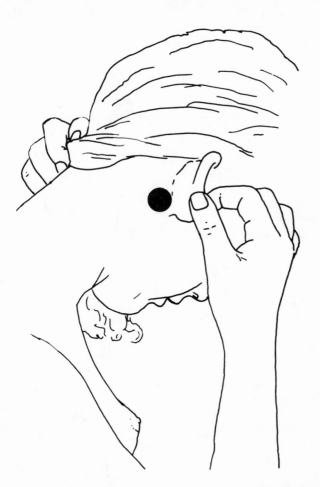

G-Jo Point No. 89

Directly behind the lower part of the ear, in the hollow where neck, jaw and ear come together.

TYPE 1

Colds and influenza
Ear, especially if painful and/or damp and
    itchy
Hearing difficulties
Tinnitus

TYPE 2

Deafness, temporary, partial
Facial paralysis, temporary
Mumps

G-Jo Point No. 90

The width of two thumbs above the top of the ear, in line with the rearward half of the ear, on the skull.

TYPE 1

Eye

TYPE 2

Intoxication; to help relieve problems after the intoxication has passed; not to be used during intoxication

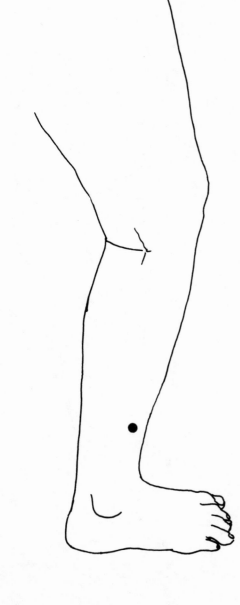

G-Jo Point No. 91

The width of one hand above the crown of the *outer* ankle, slightly forward of directly above the ankle.

TYPE 1

Diarrhea

TYPE 2

Appendicitis, acute
Beriberi
Dysentery
Fear control center
Temper control center

G-Jo Point No. 94

Between the ninth and tenth ribs (from the top of the ribcage), directly beneath the nipples.

This point has no Type 1 use.

TYPE 2

Childbirth, to help a difficult delivery; and for postpartum difficulties
Hypertension (high blood pressure)
Liver
Peritonitis

G-Jo Point No. 95

The width of one hand and one thumb above the navel, along the mid-line.

TYPE 1

Abdomen, upper
Colic
Constipation
Diarrhea, plus no. 9
Indigestion
Stomach
Vomiting, plus no. 9

TYPE 2

Cholera
Dysentery
Hiccoughs (hiccups) control center
Hypertension (high blood pressure)
Irrationality, temporary
Paralysis, temporary

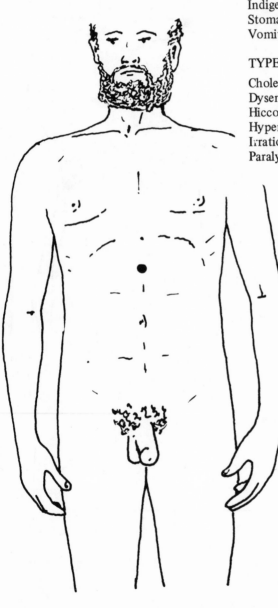

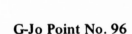

G-Jo Point No. 96

The width of two thumbs below the
bottom of the breastbone (sternum,
below the xiphoid process), along the
mid-line.

TYPE 1

Colic
Indigestion

TYPE 2

Bronchitis
Epileptic seizures
Fear control center
Hiccoughs (hiccups) control center
Malaria
Mental disturbances, temporary
Peritonitis
Pleurisy

G-Jo Point No. 97

In the center of the breastbone (sternum), in line with the nipples (must be compensated for in the case of an adult female).

TYPE 1

Bronchitis
Cough
Fatigue
Insomnia
Respiratory system

TYPE 2

Bioenergy control center
Breasts
Exhaustion
Fear control center
Head injuries; plus no. 105, if death
    seems imminent
Hiccough (hiccups) control center
Lungs
Restlessness
Sleep control center
Smoking control center

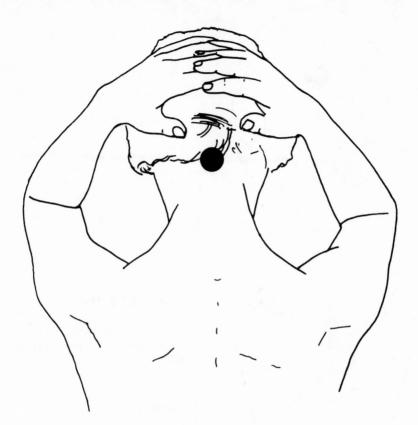

G-Jo Point No. 98

On the spine, where the spine joins the skull (cervical atlas).

TYPE 1

Colds and influenza
Headache
Hearing difficulties
Earache
Nasal congestion (catarrh)
Neck
Nosebleed (epistaxis)
Toothache

TYPE 2

Deafness, partial, temporary
Jaundice
Mental disturbances
Paralysis, half-body (hemiplegia); temporary
Suicidal actions
Vertigo

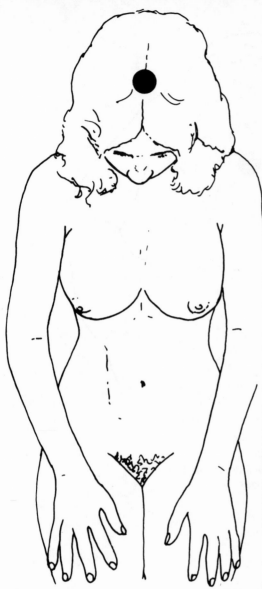

G-Jo Point No. 99

On the top of the head, midway between the ears. *Do not use this point on a small child.*

TYPE 1

Diarrhea
Eye
Flatulence
Headache
Hearing difficulties
Hemorrhoids
Nasal congestion (catarrh)
Nervousness
Throat

TYPE 2

Cerebral hemorrhage
Conjunctivitis
Convulsions, especially in older children
Deafness; partial, temporary
Fright, extreme
Hysteria
Mental disturbances
Paralysis, half-body (hemiplegia); temporary
Stricture of urine
Suicidal actions
Vertigo

G-Jo Point No. 100

The width of one thumb below the area where the skull joins the spine (cervical atlas), on the spine.

TYPE 1

Ear
Hearing difficulties
Neck
Nosebleed (epistaxis)

TYPE 2

Deafness; partial, temporary
Epileptic seizures

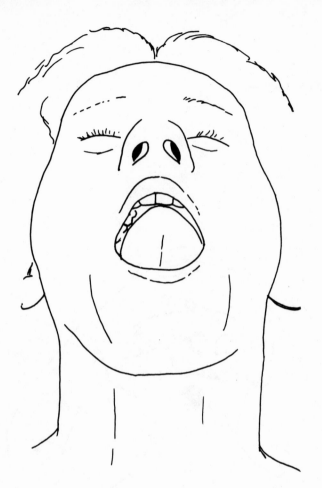

G-Jo Point No. 101

At the *outermost* portion of the inner nostril (ala nosi); at the inside flare of the nostril.

TYPE 1

Eye
Headache
Migraine

TYPE 2

Fever control center
Pain control center (eye)

G-Jo Point No. 102

Just beneath the tip of the tongue, *right side only*, toward the base or root.

TYPE 1

Sores in mouth

TYPE 2

Thirst control center

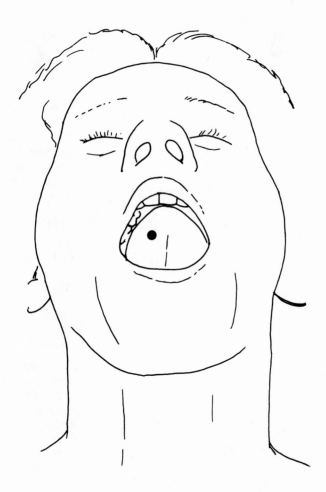

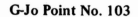

G-Jo Point No. 103

Between the neck and the tip of the
shoulder, slightly closer to the arm, and
just to the rear of the top of the muscle
stretching from the neck to the shoulder
(trapezius).

TYPE 1

Arm
Back, upper
Bruises
Elbow
Neck
Shoulder

TYPE 2

Head injuries
Hemorrhage, plus no. 20, followed in ten
    minutes by no. 21
Hypertension
Shock
Warm-up control center; to stimulate a
    feeling of warmth and to increase
    circulation

G-Jo Point No. 104

On the top of the foot, midway between
where the foot joins the leg and the toes,
in line with the second toe.

TYPE 1

Foot
Neck
Shoulder

TYPE 2

Fever control center
Poisoning, food; if severe, plus no. 18 or
    no. 105

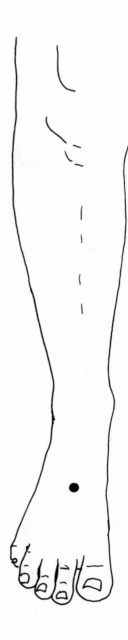

G-Jo Point No. 105

The width of two thumbs above and in line with, the nipples. *This point should not be used on a female.*

TYPE 1

Heartburn

TYPE 2

Breath control; to be used immediately before the need to breathe deeply and hard

Head injuries, plus no. 97, when death seems imminent

Poisoning, food; plus no. 104, each half hour

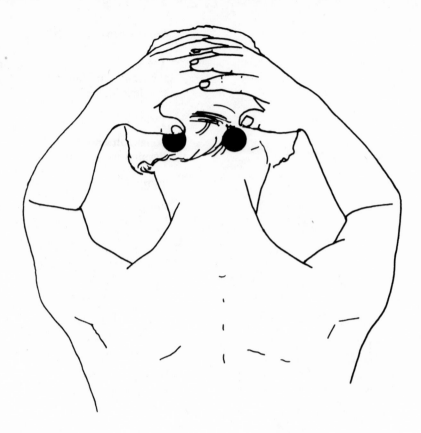

G-Jo Point No. 106

On the back of the neck, the width of two thumbs to either side of the point where the skull joins the spine (cervical atlas).

TYPE 1

Eyes
Headache
Hearing difficulties
Hives and rash (urticaria)
Migraine
Nasal congestion (catarrh)
Neck
Nosebleed (epistaxis)
Shoulder
Tinnitus
Toothache

TYPE 2

Breasts
Conjunctivitis
Deafness, temporary, partial

G-Jo Point No. 107

The width of one thumb to either side of
the spine, in line with the top of the
shoulder blades.

TYPE 1

Cough, plus no. 18
Respiratory system

TYPE 2

Lungs
Pneumonia

G-Jo Point No. 108

On the back of the skull, the width of
one hand above the base of the skull
(cervical atlas), in line with the top of the
ears.

TYPE 1

Flatulence
Indigestion

TYPE 2

Hypoglycemia (low blood sugar)
Stamina control center; to temporarily
   increase stamina

G-Jo Point No. 109

The width of one thumb to either side of the spine, on a line the width of one hand above a line between the elbows.

This point has no Type 1 use.

TYPE 2

Diabetes (diabetes mellitus)
Jaundice
Pancreas
Spleen

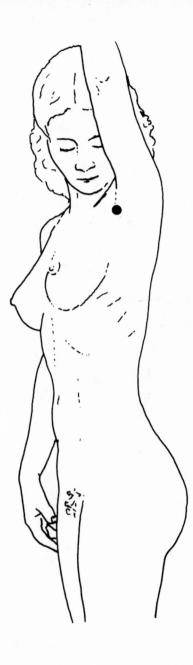

G-Jo Point No. 110

In the armpit, against the highest rib reached with a moderate fingertip probe.

This point not for Type 1 use.

TYPE 2

Bleeding, arterial; *left side only*
Bleeding, venous; *right side only*
Hypotension (low blood pressure)
Thirst control center

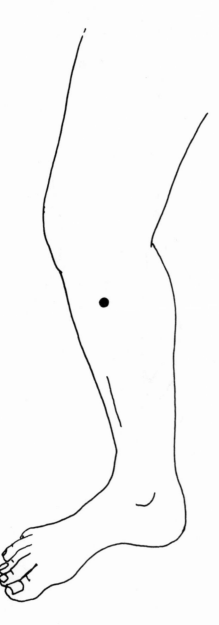

G-Jo Point No. 111

The width of one hand and two thumbs below the bottom of the kneecap, just behind the bone (tibia, "shin bone") on the *inner* leg.

This point has no Type 1 use.

TYPE 2

Bleeding, anywhere in body
Drug abuse
Hemorrhage
Lumbago
Sexual organs

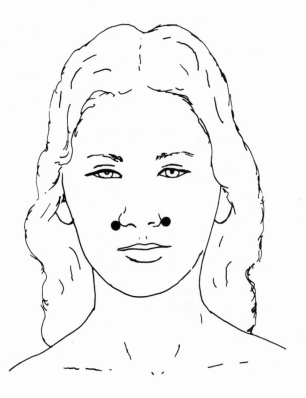

G-Jo Point No. 112

At the flare of the outer nostrils where they join the cheek; on the cheek, rather than on the nostrils.

TYPE 1

Allergies
Bronchitis
Colds and influenza
Nasal congestion (catarrh)
Respiratory system
Sinusitis

TYPE 2

For more serious problems associated with Type 1 symptoms.

G-Jo Point No. 113

The width of one hand in front of, and slightly below, the canal of the ear, atop the cheekbone prominence.

TYPE 1

Eye
Toothache

TYPE 2

Infection

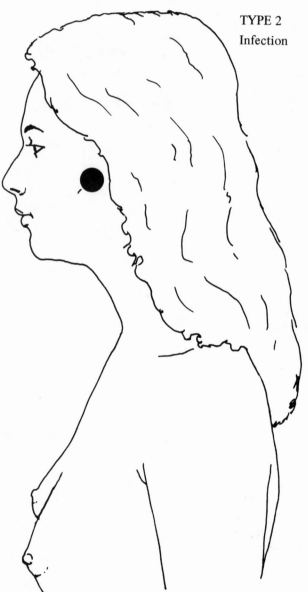

G-Jo Point No. 114

The width of three thumbs away from the crown of the *outer* ankle, in a line drawn between the crown of the outer ankle and the nail of the smallest toe.

TYPE 1

Backaches
Bladder, urinary
Herpes simplex virus
Shingles

TYPE 2

For more serious problems associated
   with Type 1 symptoms.

G-Jo Point No. 115

Midway between the nose and the upper lip.

TYPE 1

Allergies
Cramps, muscular; nocturnal leg
   cramps
Frigidity
Migraine
Toothache

TYPE 2

Drowning
Edema
Electric shock (electrocution)
Fainting
Hunger control center
Shock
Sneezing control center
Unconsciousness

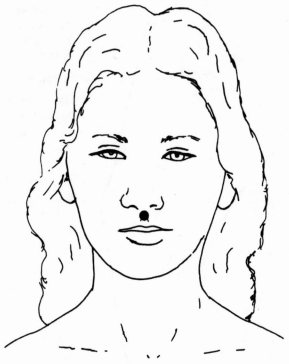

G-Jo Point No. 116

The width of two thumbs below
the end of the crease (top of the
arm) at the elbow, in line with
the middle finger.

TYPE 1

Arm
Back, upper
Bursitis
Forearm
Hand
Neck
Pain, loin to navel
Shoulders
Toothache
Wrist

TYPE 2

Shock
Unconsciousness
Whiplash

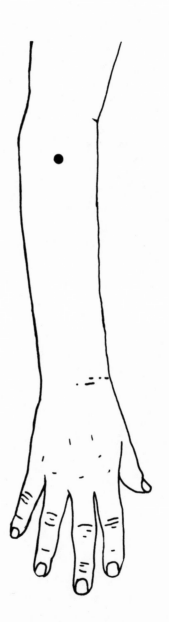

Those titles keynoted below with a double asterisk (**) may be of particular interest to medical people, while those with a single asterisk (*) are more general in their appeal.

*   *Acupuncture Anaesthesia.* Peking, China: Foreign Languages Press, 1972.
*   American National Red Cross, The. *First Aid Textbook.* New York: Doubleday & Co., Inc., fourth edition, 1971.
** Austin, Dr. Mary. *Acupuncture Therapy.* New York: ASI Publishers, Inc., 1972.
*   *Barefoot Doctor's Manual, A* (N.I.H. 75-695) Superintendant of Documents, Washington, D.C. 20402.
*   Beau, Georges. *Chinese Medicine.* New York: Avon Books, 1972.
*   *Blakiston's Pocket Medical Dictionary.* New York: McGraw-Hill Book Co., third edition, 1973.
*   Chan, Pedro. *Finger Acupressure.* Los Angeles: Price/Stern/Sloan Publishers, 1974.
*   Chan, Pedro. *Wonders of Chinese Acupuncture.* Alhambra, CA: Borden Publishing Co., 1973.
*   Duke, Marc. *Acupuncture.* New York: Pyramid Books, 1972.
*   *Emergency Care and Transportation of the Sick and Injured.* Chicago: American Academy of Orthopaedic Surgeons, 1971.
** Hashimoto, Mme. Dr. M. *Japanese Acupuncture.* 91 St. Martins Lane, London W.C.2, England: Thorson's Publishers, Ltd., 1962.
*   Houston, F.M., D.C. *The Healing Benefits of Acupressure.* New Canaan, CT.: Keats Publishing, Inc., 1974.
** Huang, Helena L., Ph.D. (translator) *Ear Acupuncture.* Emmaus, PA: Rodale Press, 1974.
*   Jain, K.K., M.D. *The Amazing Story of Health Care in China.* Emmaus, PA: Rodale Press, 1973.
** Kao, Frederick F., editor. *The American Journal of Chinese Medicine.*, Volumes I, II, III, through number 3, July, 1975.
** Lavier, Dr. J. *Points of Chinese Acupuncture (translated, indexed, and adapted by Dr. Philip M. Chancellor).* Denington Estate, Wellingborough, Northhamptonshire, England: Health Science Press, second edition, 1974.

* Lawson-Wood, D. & J. *Acupuncture Handbook.* England: Health Science Press, second edition, 1973.

* Lawson-Wood, D. & J. *First Aid at Your Fingertips.* England: Health Science Press, 1963.

** Lawson-Wood, D. & J. *Five Elements of Acupuncture and Chinese Massage.* England: Health Science Press, 1966.

* Lawson-Wood, D. & J. *Judo Revival Points, Athletes' Points and Posture.* England: Health Science Press, 1960.

* Lawson-Wood, D. & J. *The Incredible Healing Needles.* England: Health Science Press, 1974.

* Manaka, Dr. Y., and Urquhart, Dr. I.A. *Chinese Massage.* San Francisco: Japan Trading Co., 1973.

** Mann, Felix, M.B. *Acupuncture, the Ancient Chinese Art of Healing.* London: Wm. Heinemann Medical Books, Ltd., second edition, 1971.

* Mann, Felix, M.B. *Acupuncture, the Ancient Chinese Art of Healing and How It Works Scientifically.* New York: Vintage Books (division of Random House), 1973.

* Mann, Felix, M.B. *Acupuncture, Cure of Many Diseases.* London: Wm. Heinemann Medical Books, Ltd., 1971.

** Mann, Felix, M.B. *Atlas of Acupuncture.* London: Wm. Heinemann Medical Books, Ltd., 1971.

** Mann, Felix, M.B. *The Meridians of Acupuncture.* London: Wm. Heinemann Medical Books, Ltd., 1971.

** Mann, Felix, M.B. *The Treatment of Disease by Acupuncture.* London: Wm. Heinemann Medical Books, Ltd., second edition, 1967.

** Matsumoto, Teruo, M.D., Ph.D., F.A.C.S. *Acupuncture for Physicians.* Springfield, IL: Charles C. Thomas, Publishers, 1974.

** *Merck Manual of Diagnosis and Therapy, The.* Rahway, NJ: Merck & Co., Inc., eleventh edition, 1966.

** McGarey, Wm. A., M.D. *Acupuncture and Body Energies.* Phoenix, AR: Gabriel Press, 1974.

* Moss, Dr. Louis. *Acupuncture and You.* 2 All Saints St., London, N.1.: Elek Books, 1964.

* Manikoshi, Tokujiro. *Shiatsu.* San Francisco: Japan Publications Trading Co., 1969.

* Ohsawa, George. *Acupuncture and the Philosophy of the Far East.* Los Angeles: Tao Books, 1971.

* Ohsawa, George. *The Unique Principle.* San Francisco: Geo. Ohsawa Macrobiotic Foundation, Inc., 1973.

* Palos, Stephan. *The Chinese Art of Healing.* New York: Bantam Books, 1972.

* Serizawa, Katsusuke, Prof., M.D. *Massage, the Oriental Method.* San Francisco: Japan Trading Co., 1972.

** Silverstein, M.E., et al. *Acupuncture and Moxibustion (prepared by the Dept. of Health, Ho Pei Providence, China)*. New York: Schocken Books, Inc., 1975.

* Stiefvater, Dr. Eric H. *What is Acupuncture? How Does It Work?* England: Health Science Press, 1971.

** Thie, John F., D.C. *Touch for Health*. Santa Monica, CA: DeVorss and Co., Publishers, 1973.

** Toguchi, Masaru. *The Complete Guide to Acupuncture*. New York: Frederick Fell Publishers, Inc., 1974.

* Veith, Ilza (translated and introduced by). *The Yellow Emperor's Classic of Internal Medicine (Huang Ti Nei Ching Su Wen)*. Berkeley, CA: University of California Press, 1972.

* Wallnofer, Heinrich, and Von Rottauscher, Anna. *Chinese Folk Medicine*. New York: New American Library, Inc., 1972.

** Wei-P'ing, Dr. Wu. *Chinese Acupuncture*. England: Health Science Press, 1962.

** Wilner, R.E., M.D. *Acupuncture Desk Reference*. North Miami Beach, FL: Medical Diagnostic Institute, 1974.

Further information about G-Jo and other natural health techniques may be obtained by writing:

The G-Jo Institute
P.O. Box 8060
Pembroke Pines, FL 33023